HEPATOLOGY RESEARCH AND CLINICAL DEVELOPMENTS

LIVER DISEASE AND PERITONITIS

CAUSES, TREATMENT AND PREVENTION

HEPATOLOGY RESEARCH AND CLINICAL DEVELOPMENTS

Additional books in this series can be found on Nova's website under the Series tab.

Additional E-books in this series can be found on Nova's website under the E-book tab.

HEPATOLOGY RESEARCH AND CLINICAL DEVELOPMENTS

LIVER DISEASE AND PERITONITIS

CAUSES, TREATMENT AND PREVENTION

MAO KANG VOUNG
AND
JIANG SHI SUNG
EDITORS

Nova Biomedical Books
New York

For permission to use material from this book please contact us:
Telephone 631-231-7269; Fax 631-231-8175
Web Site: http://www.novapublishers.com

NOTICE TO THE READER

Library of Congress Cataloging-in-Publication Data

Liver disease and peritonitis : causes, treatment, and prevention / editors, Mao Kang Voung and Jiang Shi Sung.
p. ; cm.
Includes bibliographical references and index.
ISBN 978-1-61942-080-9 (hardcover)
I. Voung, Mao Kang. II. Sung, Jiang Shi.
[DNLM: 1. Liver Diseases--complications. 2. Peritonitis. W]

616.3'62--dc23

2011042524

Published by Nova Science Publishers, Inc. † New York

Contents

Preface

In this book, the authors present topical research in the study of the causes, treatment and prevention of liver disease and peritonitis. Topics discussed include abnormal circulating adiponectin levels which are closely associated with the development of chronic liver disease; systemic immuno-inflammatory response to severe peritonitis; the pathogenesis and therapy of peritonitis in cirrhosis; ethnic disparities in liver diseases and alteration of adhesion molecules expression and cellular polarity in liver disease. (Imprint: Nova Biomedical).

Chapter 1 – Infectious complications leading to peritonitis and, eventually, sepsis continue to be major problem in surgery. Peritonitis is an inflammation of the peritoneum from any cause. In some patients, e.g. those with necrotizing pancreatitis, enteric bacteria may infect an aseptic inflammation while in others an intra-abdominal infection is the primary cause. In infected patients with peritonitis translocation of bacteria from the gut to lymph or portal blood could be an important mechanism for the development of severe sepsis and multiple organ dysfunction syndrome (MODS).

Chapter 2 – Non-alcoholic fatty liver disease (NAFLD) is the metabolic consequence of obesity and metabolic syndrome. The incidence of childhood NAFLD has significantly increased in relation to the increasing prevalence of childhood obesity and its metabolic sequelae: dyslipidemia, hypertension and type 2 diabetes mellitus. As the incidence of childhood NAFLD has increased, so too has the more severe histologic form of NAFLD known as non-alcoholic steatohepatitis (NASH). NASH, which is characterized by inflammation, ballooning degeneration, and fibrosis, may progress to chronic, irreversible liver disease or even cirrhosis during childhood. Based on current trends, NAFLD and consequently NASH are expected to become the most common causes of end-stage liver disease in both children and young adults, especially among male subjects. While the precise underlying pathophysiologic mechanism for development of NAFLD has not been identified, excessive fatty acid availability contributes to steatosis and the metabolic abnormalities associated with NAFLD. Indeed, increased adipocyte insulin resistance and lipolytic activity with marked elevation of circulating fatty acids are the likely pathogenic mechanisms leading to hepatic steatosis and, consequently, NAFLD. However, the factors influencing an individual's susceptibility for the development and progression of liver disease, such as NASH or cirrhosis, remain elusive. In addition, significant ethnic and gender differences association with the pediatric metabolic syndrome and NAFLD remain unexplained. Therefore, effective strategies are needed for identifying and treating NAFLD and preventing the progression to NASH and end stage liver disease.

Chapter 3 – Cirrhosis is the end stage liver disease and there are many complications occurring in the course of this disease. Bacterial infections are an important complication of cirrhosis and account for significant morbility and mortality. Spontaneous bacterial peritonitis (SBP) is the most common infection in cirrhosis, accounting for 25% of infections and occurs when ascites is infected; the word spontaneous indicates that infection of ascitic fluid occurs in absence of an identified intra-abdominal source of infection, unlike other form of peritonitis. The pathogenetic mechanism of SBP is a condition known as bacterial translocation (BT) defined as a migration of bacteria or their products from the gut to mesenteric lymph nodes or to other organs. In fact most of SBP is caused by Gram-negative bacteria (GNB) of intestinal origin. Through an early diagnosis and treatment, the mortality of SPB was reduced to 20%. An empirical antibiotic therapy should be initiated immediately upon diagnosis, taking into account that the main causative agents of the SBP are GNB aerobic bacteria and an antibiotic prophylaxis should be performed in any patient at risk (eg patients with digestive bleeding, patients with a previously history of SBP). This review summarizes the main knowledge about peritonitis in cirrhosis, from pathogenesis to therapy.

Chapter 4 – Chronic liver disease is a major cause of morbidity and mortality among ethnic minorities. Additionally, ethnic variations exist in liver disease prevalence, clinical presentation, therapeutic outcome, access to health care and healthcare utilization. The numerous differences are inter-related and present unique challenges that contribute to the health diversity in the multiethnic populations. This review will discuss the existing literature on ethnic variations in chronic liver diseases. It will also provide better understanding of ethnic disparities in this population, and address clinical implications of this disparity where applicable.

Chapter 5 – The expression of the adhesion molecules in normal liver tissues, benign including probable premalignant lesions, and malignant lesions was systematically investigated in the authors' previous study. In a normal liver, both hepatocytes and bile duct cells expressedtight junction proteins (ZO-1, symplekin), adherens junction proteins (E-cadherin, α-catenin, β-catenin, γ-catenin), and desmosome proteins (desmoglein 1/2, desmocollin 2, desmoplakin, and plakophilin 2), but did not express some desmosome proteinssuch as desmocollin 1/3 and plakophilin 1. In the benign hepatocyte lesions, expression of the adherens junctions and the desmosomes was uniform and slightly increased, but symplekin appeared in a reduced expression in dysplastic lesions. In hepatocellular carcinomas (HCCs), expression of the adhesion molecules was often heterogeneous and in an abnormal location. Tumor cells with an abnormal distribution or loss of adhesion molecules show an apolar arrangement oftissue architecture. The expression levels of the adhesion molecules correlated with the differentiation grades of HCC. Furthermore, the authors found that abnormal expression of symplekin was involved in the loss of cellular polarity, the increased permeability of epithelial monolayers, and the change of cellular proliferation in vitro. Alteration of adhesion molecules and cellular polarity plays pathophysiological roles in the development and progress of hepatocellular carcinomas: (1) Abnormal location and decrease/loss of the adhesion molecules in cancer cells may reduce the adherence of hepatocytes to their neighboring cells. These functions might cause or promote invasive growth of tumor cells; (2) Some adhesion molecules (e.g. ZO-1 and β-catenin) are associated with signal transduction. Abnormal expression and distribution of the adhesion molecules may interfere with normal signal transduction and cell proliferation;(3) Adhesion molecules of epithelial cells play an important role in maintaining cellular polarity. Because of loss of polarity in cancer cells due to reduction of the adherence between hepatocytes, other adhesion molecules e.g. integrins and CD44, could be located anywhere on the cell surface of apolar cancer cells instead of its restricted domain localization in normal cells and might allow aberrant binding to the extracellular matrix and endothelial cells. In addition, some adhesion moleculessuch as E-cadherin, desmoglein 1, desmoglein 2, desmocollin 2, desmoplakin, and plakophilin 2, are tightly restricted to the epithelial constituents in a normal liver and in various liver diseases, but are completely lacking in hematopoietic and endothelial cells. These epithelial cell-specific adhesion molecules could be applied as targets to detect carcinoma cells in blood or bone marrow for early detection of HCC and for prognosis of metastases.

Chapter 6 – The inflammation of the peritoneum, a mesothelial membrane, is referred to as peritonitis. The most common cause of peritonitis is bacterial contamination. The other causes are tuberculosis, Chlamydia, fungi, chemical, biliary, drugs and foreign body. Peritonitis can be differentiated into primary, secondary and tertiary. The most common symptom with which the patient presents is pain which can be localized or generalised. Associated symptoms may include anorexia, nausea, vomiting and malaise. Patients may also present with systemic inflammatory response with fever, tachycardia and tachypnoea. Some patients may present in septic or hypovolemic shock. Tenderness, guarding and rebound tenderness are present on abdominal examination. Bowel sounds are either diminished or absent. The aim of the treatment is to restore the fluid and electrolyte balance, provide support to the organs and control the source of infection. Initial management is to control the pain, fluid resuscitation, appropriate broad spectrum antibiotics intravenously and oxygen. Definitive management is surgery and should not be delayed except for certain cases like acute pancreatitis. Surgical treatment is mainly laparotomy, though it may be possible to manage some cases by laparoscopy. The aim is to control the source of infection by resection or closure, draining abscesses, removing debris and necrotic tissues by lavage or debridement. Most cases of peritonitis cannot be prevented. It is possible to reduce the incidence of peritonitis in specific cases. Long term antibiotic prophylaxis is proven to reduce the incidence of spontaneous bacterial peritonitis in patients with cirrhosis. Incidence of peritonitis can be reduced in patients on continuous ambulatory dialysis by measures to prevent the invasion of bacteria through or around the lumen of the catheter. Taking steps to avoid the rupture of dermoid cyst during surgery will prevent cases of chemical peritonitis.

In: Liver Disease and Peritonitis
Editor: Mao Kang Voung et al.
ISBN 978-1-61942-080-9

Chapter 1

Systemic Immuno-Inflammatory Response to Severe Peritonitis

Maja Surbatovic and Nikola Filipovic
Clinic of Anesthesiology and Intensive Therapy
Military Medical Academy, Belgrade, Serbia

Infectious complications leading to peritonitis and, eventually, sepsis continue to be major problem in surgery. Peritonitis is an inflammation of the peritoneum from any cause. In some patients, e.g. those with necrotizing pancreatitis, enteric bacteria may infect an aseptic inflammation while in others an intra-abdominal infection is the primary cause. In infected patients with peritonitis translocation of bacteria from the gut to lymph or portal blood could be an important mechanism for the development of severe sepsis and multiple organ dysfunction syndrome (MODS).

Although sepsis is generally associated with a high mortality, patients with septic peritonitis have a particularly high mortality rate of 60-80%. Septic peritonitis is characterized by peritoneal mesothelial cell activation, massive infiltration of neutrophils and macrophages into the peritoneum where these cells are the first line of defense for clearing invading microorganisms. However, once they fail to restrict microbes to the peritoneal cavity, microbes may reach systemic circulation, resulting in an overwhelming systemic immune response via production of inflammatory mediators such as proinflammatory and anti-inflammatory cytokines. Such mediators in turn play a key role in the pathogenesis of septic shock and MODS.

The inflammatory response contributes significantly to the morbidity and mortality of critically ill patients and displays high level of interindividual variation. There is tremendous variability seen in the clinical profile and outcome in patients who encounter similar infective insults. Despite significant advances in understanding of the biology of inflammation, improvements in clinical outcomes have been more sporadic and, with few notable exceptions, are related to improvements in supportive care rather than to specific therapies. As a result, morbidity, mortality and cost remain high. Therefore, focus of research has more recently shifted to identification of genetic determinants of the inflammatory response in generalized peritonitis, among other conditions, especially to the group of genes that regulates immune response to infection.

Anatomy of the Peritoneal Membrane

Anatomically, the peritoneal membrane consists of two layers: 1) a squamous epithelial-like monolayer, known as the mesothelium, and 2) its underlying connective tissue. These two layers are separated from each other by an intervening basement membrane. One of the best and most concise reviews of peritoneal membrane anatomy and physiology from clinical point of view was performed by Nagy and Jackman [1]. The mesothelium, covering both the parietal and the visceral surfaces of the peritoneal membrane, consists of a single cell type, the peritoneal mesothelial cell (PMC). The number of PMCs covering the peritoneal membrane is quite large (i.e. ~ 1×10^9 PMCs cover the ~ 1-2 m^2 peritoneal surface area in man). Therefore, PMCs are one of the most numerous resident cell types within the peritoneal membrane. Mesothelium has a characteristic mosaic pattern. Ultrastructural analysis of the individual PMCs reveals numerous apical surface microvilli, a prominent rough endoplasmatic reticulum, intracellular pinocytotic vesicles, and a number of intracellular as well as extracellularly-associated lamellar bodies. Lamellar bodies produce surfactant. Besides acting as lubricants, surfactant-like materials composed of phospholipids work synergistically with complement. For example, they work together as opsonins to promote the phagocytosis of bacteria, and have a protectant role at mucosal, serosal and synovial surfaces. Both cell-cell and cell-matrix interactions contribute to the structural integrity of the mesothelium. Individual MCs are sealed together into an epithelium-like sheet by tight junctions; anchoring junctions (AJs), composed of adherens junctions and desmosomes, attach PMCs to their neighbors or to the underlying basement membrane; gap junctions (GJ) mediate the passage of chemical or electrical signals from one MC to another. The MC monolayer is supported by underlying basement membrane. This thin laminar network contains type IV collagen, proteoglycans and glycoproteins such as laminin. This basal lamina is though to be produced by the MCs.

The connective tissue proper lies beneath the mesothelium and its basal lamina. This region is made up of a complex network of extracellular matrix (ECM) macromolecules consisting of collagen, elastin and fibronectin, as well as a hydrated gel composed of various glycosaminoglycans (i.e., hyaluronan, sulphated proteoglycans). Large and small caliber blood vessels can be found throughout the peritoneal membrane ECM. Draining lymphatics are located predominantly within the interstitium of the subdiaphragmatic peritoneal membrane, whereas extracellular fluid can be found throughout the ECM. In addition, various cellular elements (e.g., fibroblasts, resident tissue macrophages, and mast cells) are also interspersed within the connective tissue proper.

Physiology of the Peritoneal Membrane

The mesothelium participates in many ways to maintain the physiological homeostasis of the peritoneal cavity. To facilitate movement of opposing tissues and organs within the peritoneal cavity during peristalsis and respiration, PMCs express numerous microvilli and produce lubricants, such as hyaluronic acid, and small dermatan sulfate proteoglycans, such as decorin and biglycan, as well as lamellar bodies containing phosphatidylcholine. The functional surface area of the mesothelium is increased by these numerous microvilli, which entrap the lubricants and thereby decrease surface friction [1].

Also, the mesothelium is one of several barriers to the transport of small and large solutes across the peritoneal membrane from the capillary lumen to the peritoneal cavity, although the mesothelium is not considered to offer significant resistance to such transport. Macromolecular transport across the mesothelium occurs, at least in part, by passive diffusion through intercellular clefts. However, mesothelium may actively participate in transperitoneal passage of solutes via numerous PMC plasmalemmal vesicles [1].

The normal, intact mesothelium has been shown to possess significant inherent fibrinolytic activity, which is believed to prevent the formation of fibrous adhesions between the visceral and parietal surfaces via two types of plasminogen activators, i.e., tissue plasminogen activator (t-PA) and urokinase type plasminogen activator (u-PA). Conversely, the mesothelium is also capable of secreting fibrinolytic inhibitors. In vitro, PMCs can synthesize both type 1 and type 2 plasminogen activator inhibitors (PAI-1 and PAI-2) as well as other anti-plasmins.

PERITONEAL MESOTHELIAL cells play a central role in the biology of the peritoneal cavity, a role that extends beyond the provision of mechanisms that allow for the easy gliding of opposed peritoneal surfaces. PMCs have the same mesodermal origin as the endothelial cells that line blood vessels, and both types of cell can express specific surface markers that enable them to promote the margination and migration of neutrophils, to interact with extracellular matrix proteins, to present antigens to immune cells and to produce biologically important molecules such as inflammatory cytokines, nitric oxide, growth factor, tissue plasminogen activator and plasminogen activator inhibitor [2].

Fluid within the peritoneal cavity moves cephalad in response to pressures generated by the diaphragm. It is then absorbed into lymphatic lacunae that lie beneath gaps (stomata) in the mesothelium lining the undersurface of the diaphragm. The lymph then flows into the main lymphatic ducts via the substernal lymph nodes. It only takes a few minutes for this process to start clearing contaminants from the peritoneal cavity; the process is facilitated by stomata that are also present in the omental, mesenteric and pelvic peritoneum. The size of stomata is controlled by actin filaments and their size has been observed to increase during inflammation, from 4-10 μm to more than 20 μm. The uneven distribution of stomata within the abdomen indicates that the peritoneal mesothelium is morphologically and functionally heterogeneous. For example, PMCs covering the liver and spleen are more substantial than those overlying the intestines, omentum and parietal regions. The former are cubic cells with a cytoplasm rich in organelles, a dense microvillous coat and elaborate intercellular contacts. The latter have scant cytoplasm, few organelles and sparsely distributed microvilli. Hence, mesothelium overlying parenchymal organs have strong structural integrity as well as an inherent ability to promote the flow of fluid within peritoneal cavity by the action of the microvilli. The microvilli, which are up to 3 μm in length, project from the apical surface of PMCs and serve also to minimize the shear between neighboring peritoneal surfaces. The peritoneal mesothelium can adapt to insults. It seems that evolutionary pressures have optimized survival during peritonitis by combining the systemic removal of peritoneal contaminants with concomitant local actions designed to neutralize and localize the contaminants. The host's ability to survive peritonitis without surgical intervention relies heavily on it being able to localize the source of contamination. This is far more difficult for the host to achieve if there is a large volume of contamination. There are tangible consequences of having highly efficient clearance mechanism within the peritoneal cavity. It explains the rapid onset of systemic signs of peritonitis and it is little wonder that faecal peritonitis has such a high mortality rate when it is appreciated that the contents of the peritoneal cavity are being rapidly pumped into the systemic circulation, exposing affected patients to the problems that accompany severe sepsis [2].

Response of the Peritoneal Membrane to Injury

Normally, the mesothelium is a quiescent population of cells with a low endogenous turnover rate. Although the mesothelium is designed to withstand the sheer forces generated by movement of opposing viscera and parietal surfaces, PMCs can be removed very easily by wetting or drying, as often occurs during surgical manipulation. Following such denudation, the percentage of PMCs undergoing mitosis has been reported to increase from less than ~ 3% to as much as ~ 18% and the mesothelial repair process becomes activated. Mesothelial regeneration following simple PMC removal has been analyzed using a number of animal models. As soon as 30 min after PMC denudation, neutrophils and macrophages enter the peritoneal cavity and begin to cover the exposed basement membrane. Within 24 hr after PMC removal, the number of neutrophils decreases and the number of macrophages increases, such that by 48 hr after injury, most of the wound surface is covered by a single layer of macrophages. By 3-4 days after injury, small islets of primitive PMCs (i.e., flattened PMCs studded with short microvilli) begin to appear interspersed throughout the wound surface. Thereafter, the number of macrophages diminishes, such that by 7 – 10 days, a new intact PMC monolayer, resting on a continuous basement membrane, has completely reconstituted the denuded area [3].

PMC denudation coupled with damage to the submesothelial basement membrane and the underlying connective tissue constitutes a more complex form of acute peritoneal membrane injury. Different types of experimental treatments (e.g., tissue abrasion, crush injury, electrocautery and surgical excision) have been used to study the repair process following this type of injury. In addition to the influx of neutrophils and macrophages, such severe trauma to the peritoneal membrane is accompanied by an increase in vascular permeability (mediated by histamine released from degranulated mast cells or by actual vessel rupture) and exudation of plasma proteins, in particular fibrinogen, into the peritoneal cavity. The process of extravascular coagulation converts the soluble fibrinogen into an insoluble cross-linked fibrin gel, which is deposited on he injured peritoneal surface. The subsequent course of peritoneal wound repair depends not only on the nature and severity of the injury, but also on its impact on the inherent fibrinolytic properties of the mesothelium. If normal peritoneal fibrinolysis proceeds, healing follows a pattern similar to that described previously; i.e., macrophages remove debris within the injured peritoneal membrane and PMCs repopulate the peritoneal surface and reestablish the basal lamina. In addition, any damaged connective tissue is repaired by proliferating fibroblasts. However, if the normal peritoneal fibrinolytic activity is suppressed, and fibrin matrix is allowed to persist, it can form a bridge between two opposing injured peritoneal surfaces. This fibrin bridge is then gradually replaced by vascularized adhesions, which can permanently seal the two opposing peritoneal surfaces together. The development of such intraperitoneal adhesions can result in pathophysiological consequences such as bowel obstruction [3]

The normal peritoneal cavity contains only a small scattering of cells that include macrophages, neutrophils and lymphocytes; there are also desquamated PMCs and dendritic cells [4]. When faced with a peritoneal insult, these cells interact or cross-talk with PMCs and cells in the submesothelium, such as mast cells and fibroblasts, and become upregulated [5]. PMCs play a central role in these cell-signaling pathways and are themselves a potent source of a variety of proinflammatory mediators including interleukin (IL) -6, IL-8, monocyte chemoattractant protein (MCP)-1, macrophage inflammatory protein 1α and tumor necrosis factor (TNF)-α.

From Immune Response to Secondary Peritonitis to Severe Sepsis, Septic Shock and Multiple Organ Dysfunction Syndrome

Peritonitis means that there is inflammatory episode in peritoneal cavity regardless of cause. Sterile peritonitis can arise from the presence of blood, bile, gastrointestinal enzymes, or foreign bodies (e.g., starch) in the peritoneal cavity. But, clinically much more important is secondary peritonitis because it continues to cause high morbidity and mortality, from 30% to 90% in patients with associated severe sepsis, septic shock and multiple organ dysfunction syndrome (MODS). Secondary peritonitis is defined as peritoneal inflammation that follows intra-abdominal lesions such as anastomotic leakage, perforation of hollow viscus, and bowel necrosis, penetrating infectious or cancerous processes. Subsequent microbial contamination of the abdominal cavity leads to infection, which initiates the innate immune response. The primary host response to the invading microorganisms will be initiated by resident peritoneal macrophages and PMCs that are responsible for the primary phagocytosis and subsequent activation and recruitment of polymorphonuclear granulocytes and monocytes into the peritoneal cavity [6]. Monocytes will rapidly differentiate, increasing the macrophage population [7].

Various soluble and membrane-bound factors mediate the concerted actions, which constitute the innate response to infections and tissue damage. Cytokines are potent, low molecular weight proteins produced by nucleated cells, particularly those of the immune system, which exert control over the duration and amplitude of the immune/inflammatory response. They have a central role in positive and negative regulation of immune responses and in integrating these reactions with other physiological systems such as the complement and hematopoietic systems. Many are pro-inflammatory, e.g. tumor necrosis factor (TNF)-α, interleukin (IL)-1, IL-8, high-mobility group box (HMGB)-1, others are anti-inflammatory, e.g. IL-10 and IL-1 receptor antagonist (ra) and some possess both activities, e.g. IL-6. Cytokines act by binding to specific receptors at the target cell membrane, setting off a cascade that leads to induction, enhancement, or inhibition of number of cytokine-regulated genes in the nucleus, thereby modulating the immunological activity of the cell. During peritonitis, several cytokines are secreted by reticuloendothelial cells, mesothelial cells and peritoneal macrophages [8].

Circulating levels of both pro-inflammatory and anti-inflammatory cytokines are frequently elevated in sepsis and some relate to increased mortality. They activate numerous cellular processes and other inflammatory mediators that contribute to organ dysfunction. When microorganisms bind to phagocytic cells through surface TOLL-like receptors (TLRs), so called because they are homologues of the Drosophila protein Toll, a series of intracellular events is initiated that result in the release of cytokines. There are several forms of these receptors with TLR-2 preferentially recognizing Gram-positive bacterial toxins, for example peptidoglycans and lipoteichoic acid and TLR-4 binding to the lipopolysaccharide of Gram-negative bacteria [9, 10, 11].

Tumor necrosis factor-α (TNF-α) is a 17-kd polypeptide that is expressed in both membrane-bound and secreted forms. Activated monocytes and macrophages, T and NK cells synthesize TNF-α. TNF-α effects include IL-6 induction, tissue factor expression, downregulation of thrombomodulin gene expression, activation of fibrinolysis, cytotoxicity, upregulation of endothelial cell adhesion molecules, induction of NO synthase, neutrophil activation, antiviral activity, fever.

Interleukin-8 (IL-8) is a chemokine, an agent that recruits inflammatory cells to a site of injury. It is synthesized by monocytes, macrophages, neutrophils and endothelial cells. Following IL-8 stimulation, neutrophil function is stimulated, chemotaxis is promoted, adhesion molecule expression is upregulated and degranulation is enhanced.

Interferon-γ (IFN-γ) is produced by activated NK cells, Th1 cells and cytotoxic T cells. Biologic effects of IFN-γ include a role in the induction of the synthesis of IgG antibodies to bacterial polysaccharide antigens, potentiation of the activity of IL-12 and macrophage activation.

Interleukin-4 (IL-4) is molecule produced by activated T cells. Biologic properties of the molecule include stimulation and inhibition of various classes of T cells, suppression of TNF and IL-1 secretion.

Interleukin-10 (IL-10) is an 18-kd immunoregulatory cytokine. It is synthesized by monocytes, macrophages, T and B cells. Biologic effects of IL-10 include inhibition of inflammatory cytokine production by activated mononuclear cells, suppression of monocyte procoagulant activity and downregulation of the ability of monocytes to kill intracellular organisms.

Transforming Growth Factor-β (TGF-β) is a member of a family of proteins that play important roles in tissue development and repair. Most cells produce TGF-β and have receptors for the cytokine. TGF-β is produced by monocytes, macrophages and T cells. While it has pleiotropic effects that are cell type-dependent, the molecule's overall properties are anti-inflammatory.

Sepsis, Severe Sepsis, Septic Shock and Mods

Sepsis is systemic inflammatory response to infection. Approximately 10% to 15% of patients will either arrive at the hospital with a clinically important infection or develop one at some point during their hospital stay. Sepsis is reported to occur in 400 000 to 500 000 patients each year. Roughly 50% of such infections are caused by gram-negative bacteria, and of these cases, 10% to 20% may result in documented period of bacteriemia, with hemodynamic instability and organ dysfunction. Reported mortality rates are between 20% and 60% for severe cases.

Sepsis is an increasingly common cause of morbidity and mortality, particularly in critically ill patients, and its incidence has been increased for 137% during the last decade.

Definitions

The term "sepsis", in popular terms, implies a clinical and systemic inflammatory response arising from infection. It is apparent that a similar, or even identical, response can arise in the absence of infection. Therefore, phrase "systemic inflammatory response syndrome" has been proposed to describe this inflammatory process, independent of its cause.

Clinical manifestations of SIRS include, but are not limited to, more than one of the following:

a) a body temperature of $> 38^{\circ}C$ or $< 36^{\circ}C$;
b) a heart rate (HR) of > 90 beats/min;
c) tachypnea, as manifested by a respiratory rate of > 20 breaths/min or hyperventilation, as indicated by a $PaCO_2$ of < 35 mmHg (< 4,3 kPa);
d) an alteration of the white blood cell (WBC) count of > 12000 cells/mm^3, < 4000 cells/mm^3, or the presence of > 10% immature neutrophils.

These physiologic changes should represent an acute alteration form baseline in the absence of other known causes for such abnormalities, such as chemotherapy-induced neutropenia or leukopenia.

The systemic inflammatory response is seen in association with a large number of clinical conditions. Besides the infectious insults that may produce systemic inflammatory response syndrome, noninfectious pathologic causes may include pancreatitis, ischemia, multitrauma and tissue injury, hemorrhagic sock, immune-mediated organ injury, and the exogenous administration of such putative mediators of the inflammatory process as tumor necrosis factor (TNF) or other cytokines.

A frequent complication of systemic inflammatory response syndrome is the development of organ system dysfunction, including such well-defined clinical conditions as acute lung injury (acute respiratory distress syndrome – ARDS), shock, renal failure and multiple organ dysfunction syndrome.

When the systemic inflammatory response syndrome is the result of a confirmed infectious process, it is termed *sepsis*.

Infection is a microbial phenomenon characterized by an inflammatory response to the presence of microorganisms or invasion of normally sterile host tissue by those organisms.

Bacteriemia is the presence of viable bacteria in the blood. Presence of viruses, fungi, parasites and other pathogens in the blood should be described in a similar manner (i.e., viremia, fungemia, parasitemia, etc.).

Sepsis and its sequelae represent clinical and pathophysiologic continuum. The degree of severity may independently affect prognosis. Some clinically recognizable stages along this continuum that can adversely affect prognosis include the following:

Severe sepsis is defined as sepsis associated with organ dysfunction, hypoperfusion abnormality, or sepsis-induced hypotension. Hypoperfusion abnormalities include lactic acidosis, oliguria, or an acute alteration of mental status.

Sepsis-induced hypotension is defined by the presence of systolic blood pressure (BP) of < 90 mmHg or its reduction by ≥ 40 mm Hg from the baseline, in the absence of other causes for hypotension (e.g., cardiogenic shock).

Criteria for severe sepsis are:

a) $PaO_2/FiO_2 \leq 280$ (in the absence of pulmonary and cardiovascular illnesses);
b) hypoxemia ($PaO_2 < 70$ mmHg on $FiO_2 = 0{,}21$);
c) acidosis (serum lactate level > 3 mmol/L);
d) oliguria (diuresis < 30 ml/h, or 0,5 ml/kg/h for at least one hour);
e) cardiac output - CO > 4,0 L/min/m^2;
f) an acute alteration of mental status;
g) positive blood culture is not necessary.

Septic shock is a subset of severe sepsis and is defined as sepsis-induced hypotension, persisting despite adequate fluid resuscitation, along with the presence of hypoperfusion abnormalities or organ dysfunction. If hypotension lasts less than one hour and responds to conventional therapy (volume resuscitation or pharmacological support), it is the early phase of septic shock. If it lasts more than one hour in spite of adequate fluid resuscitation, and if vasopressor agents or high doses of dopamine are needed (> 6 μ/kg/h), it is refractory septic shock. Patients receiving inotropic or vasopressor agents might no longer be hypotensive by the time they manifest hypoperfusion abnormalities or organ dysfunction, yet they would still be considered to have septic shock.

Multiple organ dysfunction syndrome (MODS) is proposed to describe a pattern of multiple and progressive symptoms and signs that are thought to be pathogenically related. It emphasizes the dynamic nature of the process. The terminology *dysfunction* identifies the process as a phenomenon in which organ function is not capable of maintaining homeostasis. This process, which may be absolute or relative, can be more readily identified as a continuum of change over time (it emphasizes the dynamic nature of the process, in contrast to concept of organ *failure*, dichotomous event that is either present or absent). An example of relative organ dysfunction is found in the patient with normal cardiac output and systemic oxygen delivery who exhibits evidence of inadequate tissue oxygenation (e.g. lactic acidosis).

Multiple organ dysfunction syndrome may be described as being either primary or secondary. MODS develops by two relatively distinct, but not mutually exclusive, pathways.

Primary multiple organ dysfunction syndrome is the direct result of a well-defined insult in which organ dysfunction occurs early and can be directly attributable to the insult itself. An example of primary multiple organ dysfunction syndrome is organ dysfunction as the immediate result of trauma (e.g. blunt or penetrating abdominal trauma, pulmonary contusion, renal failure due to rhabdomyolisis, or the coagulopathy due to multiple transfusions). In primary multiple organ dysfunction syndrome, the participation of an abnormal and excessive host inflammatory response in both the onset and progression of the syndrome is not as evident as it is in secondary multiple organ dysfunction syndrome.

Secondary multiple organ dysfunction syndrome develops, not in direct response to the insult itself, but as the consequence of a host response, and is identified within the context of systemic inflammatory response syndrome. The systemic inflammatory response syndrome is also a continuous process, and describes an abnormal host response that is characterized by a generalized activation of the inflammatory reaction in organs remote from the initial insult. When due to infection, the terms sepsis and systemic inflammatory response syndrome are synonymous. Given that systemic inflammatory response syndrome/sepsis is a continuous process, multiple organ dysfunction syndrome may be understood to represent the more severe end of a variable severity of illness that characterizes systemic inflammatory response syndrome/sepsis. Thus, secondary multiple organ dysfunction syndrome usually evolves after a latent period after the inciting injury or event, and is most commonly seen to complicate severe infection like peritonitis [12, 13].

Severe sepsis and trauma complicated with multiple organ dysfunction syndrome (MODS) are leading causes of death in intensive therapy units with mortality rate exceeding 50%. Outcome is not determined only with infection or trauma, but also with intensity of immuno-inflammatory response, which is essential for host defense but uncontrolled leads to the MODS. In the pathophysiology of MODS first stage represents *the infectious insult* (if the sepsis is the case) or trauma. Host factors, adaptive and innate immunity, bacterial factors (endotoxin, exotoxin) have influence on infection development. Resistance to infection is the result of a number of host factors. The epithelial barrier provides an important first line of defense. This barrier may be breached by penetrating trauma or by alterations in mucosal defense that result from toxins or hemodynamic alterations. Then, process is coming to the second stage: *preliminary systemic response*, with febrile reaction. Principal mediators of immuno-inflammatory cascade are cytokines which regulate intensity and duration of immuno-inflammatory response to an insult. In this second stage pro-inflammatory cytokines exert their actions (tumor necrosis factor-α -TNF-α, IL-1, IL-8, IL-12, IFN-γ etc.). Third stage represents *overwhelming systemic response* in which the central role has the vascular endothelial cell dysfunction. Forth stage represents the *compensatory anti-inflammatory reaction* mediated by anti-inflammatory cytokines (IL-4, IL-10, transforming growth factor β- TGF-β, soluble TNF-α receptors, IL-1 receptors and IL-1 receptor antagonist - IL-1ra). Fifth stage represents *immunologic dissonance*, defined as an inappropriate, out-of balance response of the immunomodulatory system. If after local pro-inflammatory response systemic spillover of pro-inflammatory cytokines occurs, result is systemic inflammatory response syndrome (SIRS). If there was local anti-inflammatory response and systemic spillover of anti-inflammatory cytokines occurs, result is compensatory anti-inflammatory response syndrome (CARS). There is also mixed antagonists response syndrome (MARS) in which features of SIRS are present in a patient with CARS. One of the most important clinical consequences of systemic effects of pro-inflammatory (immunostimulation) and anti-inflammatory (immunosuppression) cytokines is the development of MODS. Complex immuno-inflammatory cascade is pathophysiological substrate of multiple organ dysfunction syndrome in surgical patients after sepsis and/or trauma. In this cascade, pro-inflammatory and anti-inflammatory cytokines play the pivotal role.

Multiple organ dysfunction syndrome is often associated with overwhelming infection and is the most frequent cause of late death in patients who survive the initial resuscitation after severe infection, surgical or accidental trauma. Patients with surgical trauma or infections exhibit alterations in hemodynamic, metabolic and immune responses that are largely orchestrated by endogenous mediators referred to as cytokines [14]. Severe inflammation may lead to acute multiple organ dysfunction syndrome and early death after injury. Augmented pro-inflammatory Th1 response can be deleterious to the patient. A lesser inflammatory response followed by excessive counter-regulatory anti-inflammatory response (CARS) may induce prolonged immunosuppressed state that can also be deleterious to the host. So, excessive anti-inflammatory Th2 response also leads to multiple organ dysfunction syndrome and higher mortality.

Extensive tissue trauma, surgical stress and general anesthesia have been shown to induce a remarkable alterations in the immune defense system, influencing the individual's susceptibility to bacterial, viral and fungal infection [15].

Severe acute diffuse peritonitis can evolve into multisystemic inflammatory state resulting in acute respiratory distress syndrome (ARDS), renal and hepatic failure, shock and death. These severe manifestations of acute peritonitis are believed to result from the local and systemic overproduction of both powerful proinflammatory and anti-inflammatory cytokines.

Some studies show that interaction between damaged autologous erythrocytes and monocytes has a major impact on the cytokine responses in humans [16]. An augmented cytokine production by the mononuclear phagocyte system may adversely affect the clinical course of injury and infections in patients who have received multiple transfusions.

Vast majority of patients with multiple organ dysfunction syndrome have acute respiratory distress syndrome (ARDS) and are mechanically ventilated. That also can affect their immune status because there is compelling evidence that protective ventilatory strategies attenuate pulmonary and systemic inflammatory responses, by addressing the underlying pathophysiology of ventilator-induced lung injury in patients with ARDS, and improve outcome. Evidence from both animal and clinical studies suggests that cyclic stretch induces changes in pro-inflammatory and anti-inflammatory gene expression. It consequently follows that mechanical forces may be immunomodulatory [17].

Among others, there is one very interesting explanation for poor outcome in patients with severe acute diffuse peritonitis with excessive pro-inflammatory and anti-inflammatory response. There are studies suggesting that there are positive associations among sustained and intense inflammatory responses and the incidence of bacterial infections. Authors hypothesized that cytokines secreted by the host during multiple organ dysfunction syndrome may indeed favor the growth of bacteria and explain the association between exaggerated and protracted systemic inflammation and the frequent development of infections [18].

However, the relationship of the absolute levels of cytokines in the serum of patients with multiple organ dysfunction syndrome after sepsis and/or trauma may vary because of baseline host factors, timing of sampling relative to the onset of sepsis or multiple organ dysfunction syndrome, high interindividual variations and methods of measurement. So, large quantities of pro-inflammatory cytokines are produced by monocytes when stimulated with bacterial products. During the course of multiple organ dysfunction syndrome, compensatory anti-inflammatory mechanisms may deactivate monocytes and lead to a state of "immunoparalysis" [19]. Finally, cytokines are called "biological cyanide capsules" if they escape the tight control mechanisms of the organism [20].

Contribution of Genes Polymorphism to Susceptibility and Outcome of Sepsis Associated with Peritonitis

The inflammatory response contributes significantly to the morbidity and mortality of critically ill patients and displays high level of interindividual variation. There is tremendous variability seen in the clinical profile and outcome in patients who encounter similar infective insults. Despite significant advances in understanding of the biology of inflammation, improvements in clinical outcomes have been more sporadic and, with few notable exceptions, are related to improvements in supportive care rather than to specific therapies. As a result, morbidity, mortality and cost remain high [21]. Therefore, focus of research has more recently shifted to identification of genetic determinants of the inflammatory response, especially to the group of genes that regulates immune response to infection.

More than 20 years ago, Sorensen conducted crucial study of almost 1000 adoptees which indicated a substantial inherited increase in the risk of premature death from severe infection. The death of biologic parent before the age of 50 resulted in relative risk of death in the adoptees of 5.81 for infections, which is the highest compared to all other cause [22]. A genetic polymorphism is an allelic variant that exists stably in a population in a frequency that cannot be accounted for by new mutations (generally > 1%). The most frequent type of polymorphism is the single-nucleotide polymorphism (SNP), which can be a substitution, a deletion or an insertion of a single nucleotide. Approximately 1 in every 300 do 500 bases of human DNA may be a SNP.

The proinflammatory cytokine tumor necrosis factor (TNF)-α is an essential component of the host immune response to insult. Guanine to adenine transition at the 308 site has been associated with variability in TNF-α secretion after various stimuli. This polymorphism results in two allele forms, one by which a guanine defines the common allele TNF1 and one by which an adenine defines the uncommon allele TNF2 [23].

Interleukin-10 is potent anti-inflammatory cytokine. Excess of IL-10 can induce immunosuppression and increase mortality. One of biallelic polymorphisms in the promoter region of the IL-10 gene is at position 1082. IL-10_{1082} polymorphism results from the substitution of guanine with adenine. Investigators focused on it's involvement in the susceptibility to and outcome of severe sepsis.

One of the most important link in understanding the molecular mechanisms of severe sepsis and septic shock has been the discovery that cluster of differentiation (CD)-14 is a receptor for a very wide range of microbial products including lipopolysaccharide (released from Gram-negative bacteria), peptidoglycans and lipoteichoic acid (constituents of Gram-positive bacteria). A genetic polymorphism has been identified inside the CD14 promoter sequence. It consists of a cytosine to thymine transition at base pair 159.

IL-1 receptor antagonist (IL-1ra) is a member of the IL-1 family that binds to the IL-1 receptor, thereby inhibiting the proinflammatory actions of IL-1α and IL-1β. Polymorphisms within the IL-1ra gene have been reported in intron 2 and contain a variable numbers of tandem repeats (VNTR) of 86 base pairs. Five alleles have been identified and include A1 (four repeats), A2 (two repeats), A3 (five repeats), A4 (three repeats) and A5 (six repeats) [24].

The aim of one of our previous studies was to determine whether distributions of TNF-α_{308}, IL-10_{1082}, $CD14_{159}$ and IL-1ra gene intron 2 genotypes in critically ill patients with sepsis are associated with outcome, underlying cause of sepsis (peritonitis, pancreatitis) or the type of infecting microorganism (Gram positive, Gram negative, mixed - Gram positive and Gram negative) [25]. Blood samples were obtained from 106 critically ill Caucasian patients. The majority of sepsis patients had peritonitis. The other major disease associated with sepsis was necrotizing pancreatitis and other causes included abscesses at other locations, pneumonia and mediastinitis. In some cases pancreatitis was associated with peritonitis. The 6-months mortality rate in our study population was 50%.

We have found that TNF-α_{308} genotype is associated with outcome with statistically high significance (p=0.008). All patients with AA genotype survived. Relative risk of death in patients with AG genotype was 3.250 and in those with

GG genotype was 1.923. Gordon with co-workers performed prospective multicentre study on 213 patients recruited from eight intensive care units (ICUs) [26]. When TNF-α_{308} genotype and allele frequences in ICU survivors and nonsurvivors were analyzed it turned out that GG genotype was more frequent in nonsurvivors (75% vs 60%), AG genotype was more frequent in survivors (35.6% vs 23.1%) as well as AA genotype (4.4% vs1.9%). So, in their study G allele was more frequent in nonsurvivors (86.5% vs 77.8%) and A allele was more frequent in survivors (22.2% vs 13.5%). Although those results did not reach satistical significance, trend was the same as in our study.

TNF-α is considered to be proximal and central cytokine in host immuno-inflammatory cascade regardless of initiating insult. One of the first studies to demonstrate association of the rare TNF2 (adenine) allele of the TNF-α promoter with outcome of severe sepsis and septic shock was performed by Mira et al. on 89 patients [27]. They concluded that TNF2 allele is strongly associated susceptibility to and death due septic shock; patients with the TNF2 allele had a 3.7-fold risk of death. Similarly, a US study (28) that looked at the occurrence of severe sepsis after trauma in 37 patients found that the A allele was associated with both occurrence of sepsis (OR 4.6, CI 1.9-10.9) and death (OR 2.7, CI 0.6-7.3). Watanabe with co-authors analyzed 150 consecutive critically ill patients recruited at admission to the intensive care unit, regardless of diagnosis, and found association between TNF-α_{308} A allele carriers and increased mortality rate [29].

Also, there are studies in which no association of TNF2 allele and increased mortality rate was found. In one of those, total of 112 postoperative critically ill infected patients were prospectively enrolled. Authors found that patients carrying the TNF2 allele were not more likely to develop septic shock, nor did they have a higher mortality rate. Only when septic shock had developed, in that subgroup of patients the mortality rate was higher in those carrying the TNF2 allele [30]. Barber with coauthors showed that TNF-α_{308} polymorphisms were significantly associated with an increased risk for severe sepsis following burn trauma but none of SNPs were significantly associated with mortality [31]. TNF-α genotype was not related to mortality in the study in which 88 critically ill patients with multiple organ dysfunction syndrome (MODS) were enrolled [32]. No significant association of any TNF-α_{308} genotype with pancreatitis as underlying cause of sepsis was found in our study. This is in accordance with findings in other studies [33, 34].

In our study, association between distribution of three IL-10_{1082} genotypes and the type of infecting microorganism is statistically highly significant (p=0.009). In patients with Gram positive sepsis AA and then AG genotypes were the most frequent ones. In patients with Gram negative sepsis GG genotype was the most frequent one. There are very few studies in literature available to us that are similar to ours in this aspect. In a review regarding genetic variability in the systemic inflammatory response only one study of IL-10_{1082} polymorphism and type of infecting microorganism in severe sepsis is mentioned: GG genotype was associated with greater risk for meningococcal disease [35]. Taking in consideration that *N. meningitidis* is Gram-negative bacterium, this is in concordance with our finding.

As far as underlying cause of sepsis (peritonitis, pancreatitis) is concerned, we found that distribution of three IL-10_{1082} genotypes is also associated with statistically high significance (p=0.003). In patients with sepsis associated with pancreatitis AA genotype was the most frequent one. In patients with sepsis associated with peritonitis GG genotype was the most frequent one. Although any genetic factor that alters the expression of regulatory cytokines-chemokines could potentially alter the inflammatory response to pancreatic injury [36], there are few studies that address this issue. One of them showed, contrary to our results, that genetic factors are not important in determination of disease severity or susceptibility to severe acute pancreatitis [37].

Comparison of IL-10_{1082} AA genotype with combination of AG and GG, showed that there is statistically significant association with outcome in our study. Critically ill patients with G allele in either of genotypes have relative risk of death 1.46; OR 2.43; 95% CI 0.894 - 6.612. Majority of other studies also demonstrated that G allele is associated with higher mortality rate [38, 39, 40]. IL-10 is one of the most important anti-inflammatory cytokines. It downregulates the production of proinflammatory cytokines and chemokines by activated monocytes, polymorphonuclear leucocytes and eosinophils, prevents antigen-specific T-cell activation, inhibits T-cell expression and potentiates the release of the inflammatory modulator IL-1ra. This IL-10 polymorphism, associated with high interleukin-10 inducibility, might influence the outcome via induced immunosuppression and impaired bacterial clearance. One study showed that allele frequencies and genotype distribution of the IL-10_{1082} polymorphism did not differ between surviving and dead patients [41] and the other, contrary to our results but in slightly different patient population (all patients developed acute respiratory distress syndrome - ARDS while in our study majority, but not all, had ARDS), showed that G allele was associated with lower mortality rate [42].

Distribution of three $CD14_{159}$ genotypes in our study showed that there is statistically significant association with the type of infecting microorganism. In patients with Gram positive sepsis CT genotype was the most frequent one. In sepsis patients with CC and TT genotypes, frequency of Gram positive and Gram negative infecting microorganisms was similar. Furthermore, we found that critically ill patients without T allele in either of genotypes i.e. with CC genotype have relative risk of Gram negative sepsis 1.25; OR 1.45; 95% CI 0.381 - 5.572. In this comparison, in sepsis patients with CC genotype Gram negative bacteria were most frequent. Contrary to our results, Sutherland with co-workers found that $CD14_{159}$ TT was associated with increased prevalence of Gram-negative bacteria in a cohort of 252 critically ill Caucasians [43] and Yuan and co-authors reported that prevalence of $CD14_{159}$ CC genotype was significantly higher in 85 children with pneumococcal (i.e. Gram-positive) sepsis [44], while, Calvano and Lowry found no association between CD14 polymorphisms and increased risk of Gram-negative infections [45].

CD14 is an innate immunity receptor for lipopolysaccharide, peptidoglycan and lipoteichoic acid. CD14 is found on the surface of monocytes, macrophages, neutrophils and hepatocytes and as a soluble form in serum. Transition of C to T at position 159 in the promoter of the CD14 gene has been associated with increased density of membrane-bound CD14 on monocytes and increased serum levels of soluble CD14. This may alter host recognition and clearance of pathogens.

We found no significant association of any CD14 polymorphism with outcome, same as Hubacek [46] and Nakada and co-workers [47]. But, some authors reported significant association of TT genotype with higher mortality rate in patients with severe sepsis and septic shock [48] and significant association of C allele with decreased risk of multiple organ dysfunction and sepsis in major trauma patients [49].

We analyzed distribution of six IL-1ra gene intron 2 genotypes, and no significant association of any genotype with underlying cause of sepsis (peritonitis, pancreatitis), with the type of infecting microorganism or with outcome was found. Similar findings reported Powell [34] who also found no association of IL-1ra polymorphism with pancreatitis and Fang [50] who found no association with outcome in 93 patients with severe sepsis.

IL-1ra is a naturally occurring competitive inhibitor of interleukin-(IL)-1 induced proinflammatory activity. The IL-1ra gene is polymorphic, resulting in quantitive differences in IL-1ra production. The relative levels of IL-1ra and IL-1 at an inflammatory site will determine whether a proinflammatory response will be initiated and persist or will be terminated. Persons homozygous for allele 2 of the IL-1ra gene have a more prolonged and more severe proinflammatory immune response than persons with other IL-1ra genotypes because they produce significantly lower levels of IL-1ra [51]. There are studies in which significant association between A2/A2 polymorphism and higher mortality rate was demonstrated in patients with severe sepsis [52, 53].

Evidently, there are inconsistent findings in current studies of genetic associations in human trauma and/or sepsis. Strict critics attribute that to methodological and analytical problems (underpowered studies, inadequate size of the study etc.) but they also state that, for example, it has been calculated for a general ICU population with sepsis or septic shock, a sample size of 2000 patients would be required to detect a mortality relative risk of 1.5 from any polymorphism to confidently exclude false negative associations. To our knowledge no genetic association study recruited this number of patients. Until then, relatively small population studies should be taken in to account.

Although most studies are of small more or less homogeneous populations, the identification of strong associations between certain genetic polymorphisms and increased mortality rate, underlying cause of sepsis or the type of infecting microorganism is intriguing and supports further research using this approach. The establishment of these associations does not equal causation, and further research is required in both genetic and molecular aspect of host immuno-inflammatory response to various insults in critically ill patients. Examination of the association between genetic polymorphisms and sepsis regardless of underlying cause, peritonitis for example, promises to provide clinicians with new tools to evaluate prognosis, to intervene early and aggressively in treating high risk patients, and to avoid the use of therapies with adverse effects in treating low risk patients. Genomic information may be useful to identify groups of patients with high risk of developing severe sepsis and multiple organ dysfunction syndrome associated with diffuse peritonitis [54].

Infection and Inflammation in Secondary Peritonitis

In sepsis associated with secondary peritonitis, gut barrier dysfunction is common feature. Critically ill patients are susceptible to injury of the intestinal mucosa, changes in gut permeability and failure of gut-associated lymphoid tissue (GALT). Bacterial translocation is defined as the passage of viable bacteria, usually Gram-negative aerobes and/or their endotoxins from the gut lumen to normally sterile tissues such as the mesenteric lymph nodes and beyond. Billions of bacteria (400 – 500 different species) normally inhabit the gastrointestinal tract. These bacteria are believed to be critical for normal nutrition and well-being of the host. The bacteria produce and secrete many kinds of substances into the gut lumen, including small molecules called quorum-sensing signal molecules (QSMs). Quorum-sensing signal molecules are produced by many Gram-positive and Gram-negative bacteria, some of which are present in the gut. These molecules are involved in coordinating responses of bacterial populations to environmental changes as well as generating communication signals between neighboring bacteria by freely diffusing across bacterial cell membranes. In addition, QSMs modulate immune functions in the host, thereby, enhancing bacterial survival. To date many types of QSMs have been documented. Some of the earliest and best described QSMs are those belonging to the family of N-acylhomoserine lactones produced by Gram-negative bacteria. Amongst these, N-(3-oxhexanoyl)-L-homoserine lactone (3-oxo-C6-HSL or OHHL) and N-(3-oxododecanoyl)-L-homoserine lactone (3-oxo-C12-HSL or OdDHL) have been identified in pathogenic bacteria. These molecules bind to and activate transcriptional regulators in bacteria, which in turn activate virulence gene expression that controls the virulence in bacteria, and production of secondary metabolites, in a cell density-dependent manner. Moreover, these molecules can regulate biofilm formation in bacteria, which protects them from host defenses and provides enhanced resistance to antibiotics. During infection, pathogens employ various strategies to enhance survival and multiplication. Also, various environmental signals induce the expression of virulence determinants in bacteria, such as temperature, pH, osmolarity and nutrient availability. One of the most important factors determining the infection of the host is a critical cell population density sufficient to overwhelm the host immune defenses, particularly by opportunistic pathogens in the gut. In patients with sepsis, the gut barrier function is impaired. As a result, toxic substances including QSMs and/or endotoxins from both pathogenic and non-pathogenic bacteria freely enter the host systemic circulation. These circulatory substances induce and/or modulate the subsequent host inflammatory response [55].

Peritonitis can also be associated with various types of trauma, either accidental, surgical or combat injuries. Death after trauma, infection or other critical illness has been attributed to unbalanced inflammation, in which dysregulation of cytokines leads to multiple organ dysfunction and death. In one study, authors hypothesized that admission cytokine profiles associated with death would differ based on admitting diagnosis [56]. This 5-year study included patients admitted for trauma or surgical intensive care for more than 48 hours at 2 academic, tertiary care hospitals. Cytokine analysis for IL-1, IL-2, IL-4, IL-6, IL-10, IL-12, interferon-γ and TNF-α was performed using ELISA on specimens drawn within 72 hours of admission. There were 1655 patients who had complete cytokine data: 290 infected, nontrauma; 343 noninfected, nontrauma; and 1022 trauma. Among infected patients, nonsurvivors had higher median admission levels of IL-2, IL-8, IL-10 and granulocyte macrophage-colony stimulating factor; noninfected, nontrauma patients had higher IL-6, IL-8 and IL-10; and nonsurviving trauma patients had higher IL-4, IL-6, IL-8 and TNF-α. IL-4 was the most significant predictor of death and carried the highest relative risk of dying in trauma patients and IL-8 in nontrauma, noninfected patients. In infected patients, no cytokine independently predicted death. Authors concluded that cytokine profiles of certain disease states may identify persons at risk of dying and allow for selective targeting of multiple cytokines to prevent organ dysfunction and death.

We have extensive experience with combat casualties, among which vast majority sustained blunt or penetrating abdominal trauma and who developed secondary peritonitis. The aim of one of our studies was to evaluate the immune response in combat casualties (blast or explosive trauma with or without secondary sepsis) and assess the prognostic value of pro-inflammatory TNF-α and IL-8 and anti-inflammatory cytokines IL-4 and IL-10 regarding severity and outcome [57].

The study group consisted of 76 male casualties admitted to the Clinic of anesthesiology and intensive therapy, Military Medical Academy (MMA), Belgrade, Serbia. All were wounded during bombardment. In 76% cases, the moment of sustaining injury was established. Time interval between sustaining injury and admission (when the first set of blood samples was taken) was 6 hours in 61% (initial surgical treatment was administered in MMA) and 12 hours in the rest of the cases (initial surgical treatment was administered in front line hospitals). Number of casualties enrolled in this study was limited by ELISA assays availability. Group I consisted of 56 casualties with blast or explosive trauma that developed secondary sepsis confirmed with positive blood culture (trauma + sepsis group). Group II consisted of 20 casualties, selected to match Group I: with blast or explosive trauma of the same severity as in group I, but without sepsis (trauma group). Determination of trauma severity was performed using Injury Severity Score (ISS). ISS was determined using Abbreviated Injury Scale (AIS). Casualties were divided into two groups according to severity of clinical status: Systemic Inflammatory Response Syndrome - SIRS (less severe) and Multiple Organ Dysfunction Syndrome - MODS (more severe) group. Fifty five casualties developed multiple organ dysfunction syndrome (MODS), 36 died. Blood was drown on the first day of trauma. Concentrations of IL-8, TNF-α, IL-4 and IL-10 were determined in plasma using ELISA assays. Mean values of IL-8 were 230-fold, IL-10 42-fold and TNF-α 17-fold higher in trauma + sepsis group

($p<0.01$). Mean values of IL-8 were 60-fold, TNF-α 43.5-fold and IL-10 70-fold higher in MODS group ($p<0.01$). Mean values of IL-8 were 2.3-fold and IL-10 1.4-fold higher in non-survivors and TNF-α 2.2-fold higher in survivors ($p<0.01$). IL-4 had no significance as predictor of severity and outcome contrary to the results of previous study [56].

Dimopoulou with coauthors [58] focused their investigation to determine the inter-relationships between cytokine levels and physiological scores in predicting outcome in unselected critically ill patients. To this end 127 patients with wide range of admission diagnoses (medical, surgical, and multiple trauma patients) were prospectively investigated. Severity of critical illness and organ dysfunction were graded by acute physiology and chronic health evaluation (APACHE II) and sequential organ failure assessment (SOFA) scores, respectively. Blood samples were drawn on admission in the ICU to determine pro- and anti-inflammatory cytokines, including TNF-α, IL-6, IL-8 and IL-10. The main outcome measure was 28 day mortality. Overall, 88 patients survived and 39 patients died. Authors concluded that in mixed ICU patients cytokine concentrations on admission in the ICU represent independent outcome predictors in the presence of disease severity scores.

On animal model of peritonitis, tissue and time-dependent upregulation of cytokine mRNA was investigated [59]. Objective was to quantitate the course of specific cytokine mRNA expression in tissues that exhibit increasing histopathological changes in time in an animal model for the MODS. Ninety-four C57BL/6 mice were given an intraperitoneal injection of 40 μg of lipopolysaccharide (LPS), followed by zymosan at a dose of 0.8 mg/g body weight 6 days later (day 0). Six additional animals did not receive zymosan and acted as controls. At several time points after zymosan injection, 6 randomly assigned, zymosan-treated animals were killed, and their livers, lungs, spleens, and kidneys were collected. mRNA expression of TNF-α, IL-1β, IL-6, macrophage migration inhibiting factor, IL-12, interferon-γ and IL-10 was measured using a real-time reverse transcription-polymerase chain reaction assay. The injection of zymosan induced an acute peritonitis, followed by an apparent recovery. From approximately day 6 onwards, animals started to display MODS-like symptoms. During the peritonitis phase, up-regulation of cytokine mRNA was limited. During period of apparent recovery, cytokine mRNA expression strongly increased, mostly reaching its maximum at day 9 when deterioration of the clinical condition had already set in. The up-regulation of TNF-α mRNA was most pronounced, especially in the lungs and liver. Authors concluded that interventions should preferentially be targeted against multiple cytokines and, at least in this model, there may be a treatment window well after the initial challenge.

The successful management of life-threatening infection, such as diffuse peritonitis, is grounded in two principles: early and effective elimination of invasive infection, and successful reversal of systemic physiologic derangements arising through innate host response to that infection [60]. Source control can be defined as any physical intervention that is undertaken to remove or eliminate a focus of invasive infection and to restore optimal anatomic function. Four elements are crucial: a) drainage - the evacuation of a discrete focus of infected fluid through its conversion to a controlled sinus or fistula; b) debridement – the physical removal of devitalized infected tissue; c) device removal – the removal of devices or foreign bodies that have become colonized with microorganisms, and serve as a locus of ongoing microbial seeding; and d) definitive reconstructive measures – all those interventions that serve to reconstruct the damage resulting from infection or its management.

There is dilemma regarding systemic effects of planned relaparotomy in secondary peritonitis. In one study [61] hypothesis was that planned relaparotomy (PRL) has been suggested to have detrimental effects on the systemic activation of inflammatory mediators, thereby enhancing organ dysfunctions as assessed by clinical scores in secondary peritonitis. Twenty-nine patients with secondary peritonitis were included. Of that number, 11 underwent PRL and 18 obtained primary abdominal closure. Blood samples were obtained preoperatively and at 2, 6, 8, 12, 18, 24, 30, 36, 42 and 48 hours after the primary operation, then every 12th hour until day 5 and once daily until day 8. Preoperatively, the patient groups did not differ in mean age, cause of peritonitis, or clinical scores (APACHE II and SOFA). On average, 5.1 (range 3-11) lavage treatments were performed in the PRL group, with 90% of the procedures executed during the first 6 days. The PRL treatment resulted in a significantly higher need of blood components and an increased inflammatory mediator response, especially concerning coagulation factors, proinflammatory cytokines, adhesion molecules and opsonic parameters. During PRL, clinical score systems showed higher values and a delayed decline compared with primary abdominal closure treatment. Incidence of multiorgan failure, mortality and mean intensive care unit hospitalisation period were clearly more pronounced in the PRL group. Authors concluded that additional lavage treatment of secondary peritonitis resulted in an enhancement of systemic inflammatory mediator response (in particular IL-8), which may contribute to a further impairment of organ function.

Recently, IL-27 has been identified as a new bioactive member of the IL-12 cytokine family [62]. It consists of an IL-12 p40-related polypeptide, denoted

EBV-induced gene 3 (EBI3), and a novel p28 subunit with some similarities to IL-12 p35 and IL-23 p19, respectively. Over last several years, IL-27 has emerged as a pivotal cytokine in the adaptive immune system by controlling T cell-dependent immune responses. IL-27 is novel regulator that controls the magnitude of the innate immune reaction during experimental septic peritonitis with anti-inflammatory effects. One recent study shows possible key role of IL-27 in immuno-inflammatory cascade in lethal septic peritonitis [63]. The immune response to bacterial infections must be tightly controlled to guarantee pathogen elimination while preventing tissue damage by uncontrolled inflammation. Authors in their study demonstrate key role of IL-27 in regulating this critical balance. IL-27 was rapidly induced during murine experimental peritonitis induced by cecal ligation and puncture (CLP). Furthermore, mice deficient for the EBI3 subunit of IL-27 were resistant to CLP-induced septic peritonitis as compared with wild-type controls, and this effect could by suppressed by injection of recombinant single-chain IL-27. EBI3$^{-/-}$ mice displayed significantly enhanced neutrophil migration and oxidative burst capacity during CLP, resulting in enhanced bacterial clearance and local control of infection. Fact that EBI3$^{-/-}$ mice were protected from experimental septic peritonitis and that injection of recombinant IL-27 prevented such protection is of clinical relevance. Also, EBI3$^{-/-}$ mice have significantly reduced mortality upon intraperitoneal injection of live *E. coli*. IL-27 EBI3$^{-/-}$ mice had significantly reduced numbers of bacteria in the peritoneum and blood associated with an increased oxidative burst capacity of neutrophils. The fact that neutrophils produce a cytokine such as IL-27 that inhibits their influx/activation may represent an autoregulatory loop to limit neutrophil responses. Subsequent studies demonstrated that IL-27 directly suppresses endotoxin-induced production of reactive oxygen intermediates by isolated primary granulocytes and macrophages. In vivo blockade of IL-27 function using newly designed soluble IL-27 receptor fusion protein led to significantly increased survival after CLP as compared with control-treated mice. These data identify IL-27 as a key negative regulator of innate immune cell function in septic peritonitis. Data from that study suggest a major role of IL-27 in modulating influx and oxidative burst of granulocytes and elimination of bacteria during peritonitis. Thus, early IL-27 production by myeloid cells may exert a negative feedback mechanism that limits protective innate immune responses in peritonitis. In vivo blockade of IL-27 function is a novel potential therapeutic target of treatment of sepsis. That could be achieved by using a newly designed sIL-27R fusion protein. In that scenario, experimental septic peritonitis could be suppressed and mortality reduced in vivo.

In secondary peritonitis, the gastrointestinal barrier is disrupted, which leads to intra-abdominal infection caused by microbial pathogens or their products. Intra-abdominal abscesses are well known sources of recurrent or ongoing abdominal sepsis and are, therefore, an important target for prevention or elimination. During peritonitis both intra-abdominal coagulation and fibrinolysis are upregulated to a different degree, resulting in a net increase of coagulation activity. As a consequence, fibrin deposits form, which sequestrate the source of infection but also serve as a nidus for intra-abdominal abscesses. In order to prevent abscess formation, attempts were made to enhance fibrinolytic activity with recombinant tissue-type plasminogen activator (rtPA) in rats with generalized peritonitis. Experimental data suggest that fibrinolytic therapy may be effective when antibiotics are not. In one recent study [64] peritonitis was induced via intra-abdominal injection of a faeces and bacteria mixture in male Wistar rats. Surgical debridement was performed after 1 h. Next to untreated controls, animals were treated with antibiotics (ceftriaxone plus metronidazole), recombinant tissue plasminogen activator or both. Abdominal fluid samples were taken at 24, 72 and 120 h for IL-6, IL-10 and TNF-α measurements and cell counts. After 5 days the abdomen was inspected for presence of abscesses. Antibiotics did not significantly affect abscess formation. However, giving rtPA significantly reduced the number of rats with abscesses and the abscess load per rat, both in the absence and presence of concomitant antibiotic therapy. No adverse side-effects were observed and no meaningful differences in the local inflammatory response were found. In this rat model, rtPA consistently reduced abscess formation after surgical treatment of secondary peritonitis. It therefore represents a promising adjuvant to conventional therapy.

One of the most recent studies regarding secondary peritonitis was aimed to analyze if peritoneal cytokine levels can predict survival in an experimental model for peritonitis. Early identification of patients most at risk for adverse outcomes would facilitate the decision for aggressive therapy in order to maximally exploit their chance for survival. In that study [65] peritonitis was induced by intraperitoneal injection of faeces/bacteria mixture in 175 rats. Surgical debridement was performed after 1 hour. Abdominal fluid samples were taken after 24 and 72 hours for the measurement of IL-6, IL-10 and TNF-α. Surviving animals were sacrificed after 5 days and correlations between cytokine levels and survival rate were analyzed. Sixty animals died prematurely, 12 before the first sampling of cytokines. So, 48 nonsurvivors and 115 survivors were analyzed. Peritoneal cytokine levels were much higher ($p < 0.0001$) in nonsurvivors than in survivors. At 24 hours there were strong correlations between cytokine levels, especially between IL-6 and IL-10 ($r=0.93$). Peritoneal cytokines at 24 hours also discriminated between animals dying within the next 24 hours and those dying later. A strongly ($p < 0.0001$) increased mortality was observed if IL-6, IL-10 or TNF-α levels exceeded 2, 1 or 0.2 ng/mL, respectively. Receiver operating characteristic curves were promising for all 3, but IL-10 showed the best characteristics, with an area under the curve of 0.94 and 67% sensitivity at 95% specificity, obtained at a cut-off value of 1.26 ng/mL. Authors concluded that these data should generate renewed interest to examine the peritoneal cytokines as early markers for adverse outcomes in patients with secondary peritonitis. Possibly, combination of peritoneal cytokines with other markers can lead to much needed, reliable early prediction of disease severity.

Secondary peritonitis is associated with a significant cytokine response compartmentalized in the peritoneal cavity. Many studies have shown that postoperative complications are associated with increasing levels of systemic IL-6 and peritoneal TNF-α. Postoperative intraperitoneal (peritoneal) response in repeated lavage is much higher than seen in venous (systemic) response. Jansson and coauthors conducted a study focused on intraperitoneal cytokine response after major surgery [66]. Major abdominal surgery was performed in 19 patients. Preoperative systemic measurements and postoperative systemic and peritoneal measurements of C-reactive protein (CRP) and the cytokines TNF-α, IL-6 and IL-10 were performed. Significantly higher TNF-α, IL-6 and IL-10 peritoneal values were recorded compared with systemic values, whereas peritoneal CRP was significantly decreased. CRP increased significantly over time, whereas postoperative values of IL-6, IL-10 and peritoneal TNF-α decreased. Systemic TNF-α was constant over time, but values after emergent abdominal surgery showed a more extensive response. An additional effect of surgery and emergent abdominal disease was seen in increased TNF-α and IL-10 levels. Compared with systemic cytokines, peritoneal responded extensively after major surgery, indicating that measurement of peritoneal cytokines is a more sensitive method to determine postoperative inflammatory reaction because peritoneal response is faster and higher. A normal postoperative course is characterized by decreasing levels of peritoneal cytokines.

Infectious complications leading to peritonitis and, eventually, sepsis continue to be a major problem in surgery. Peritonitis is an inflammation of peritoneum from any cause. In some patients, e.g. those with necrotizing pancreatitis, enteric bacteria may infect an aseptic inflammation while in others an intra-abdominal infection is the primary cause. In infected patients with peritonitis translocation of bacteria from the gut to lymph or portal blood could be and important mechanism for the development of sepsis and MODS. Bacterial translocation is defined as the passage of enteric microorganisms across the gut mucosa to mesenteric lymph nodes (MLNs) and from there to distant sites. It was proposed that, in man, release of cytokines form the gut triggering an inflammatory response in other parts of the body may be the major mechanism by which the gut influences the outcome of sepsis. So, in peritonitis, increased production of cytokines and changes in the splanchnic cellular immune system may cause translocation of bacteria and endotoxin. One study assessed the frequency of translocation and related translocation to the immune response in patients with acute peritonitis [67]. Patients with local (LP, n=20) or generalized peritonitis (GP, n=15) were compared with controls (C, n=12). Blood was obtained preoperatively for cultures, and analyses of endotoxin and cytokines (TNF-α, IL-6, IL-10). Mesenteric lymph nodes were excised for culturing and immunohistochemistry using antibodies CD4, CD8 and CD68. Positive blood and MLN cultures were not obtained in controls. DNA typing proved bacterial translocation in one patient with local and one patient with generalized peritonitis. Thus, translocation was proven to occur in 6% patients with peritonitis. Endotoxaemia was predominantly found in the patients with generalized peritonitis. Cytokines increased during peritonitis and more so in patients with generalized peritonitis than in those with local peritonitis. More $CD8^+$ and $CD68^+$ cells were found in MLNs from LP patients than in C patients and more $CD4^+$ and $CD8^+$ cells in LP patients than in GP patients. There was no significant difference in this regard between GP and C groups. Authors concluded that bacterial translocation occurs during acute peritonitis but seems to be fairly infrequent, and that peritonitis causes significant inflammatory cellular reaction.

Last, but not least, because of relatively high mortality rate associated with generalized peritonitis, which can exceed 50%, prognostic factors are very important. Mulier and colleagues focused their attention to prognostic factors identification in this set of patients by means of univariate and multivariate analysis in a consecutive series of 96 patients [68]. Mortality was 30%. Inability to clear the abdominal infection or to control the septic source, older age, and unconsciousness were significant factors related to mortality in the multivariate analysis. Failure to control the peritoneal infection (15%) was always fatal and correlated with failed septic source control, high APACHE II score and male gender. Failure to control septic source (8%) also was always fatal and correlated with high APACHE II score and therapeutic delay. In patients with immediate source control, residual peritonitis occurred in 9% after purulent or biliary peritonitis and in 41% after fecal peritonitis (p=0.002). In patients without immediate control of the septic source, delayed control was still achieved in 100% after a planned relaparotomy (PR) strategy versus 43% after an on-demand relaparotomy (ODR) strategy (p=0.018). In the same patients, mortality was 0% in the PR group versus 64% in the ODR group (p=0.007). Early relaparotomy is related to improved septic source control. After relaparotomy for generalized postoperative peritonitis, a PR strategy is indicated whenever source control is uncertain. It also might decrease mortality in fecal peritonitis. An ODR approach is adequate for purulent and biliary peritonitis with safe septic source control.

References

[1] Nagy JA, Jackman RW. Anatomy and physiology of the peritoneal membrane. *Semin. Dial* 1998; 11:19-56.

[2] Yao V, Platell C, Hall JC. Role of peritoneal mesothelial cells in peritonitis. *Br. J. Surg.* 2003; 90:1187-94.

[3] Nagy JA, Jackman RW. Response of the peritoneal membrane to injury. *Semin. Dial* 1998; 11:242-8.

[4] Broche F, Tellado JM. Defe.nse mechanisms of the peritoneal cavity. *Curr. Opin. Crit. Care* 2001; 7:105-16.

[5] Wojta J, Kaun C, Zorn G, Ghannadan M, Hauswirth AW, Sperr WR et al. C5a stimulates production of plasminogen activator inhibitor-1 in human mast cells and basophils. *Blood* 2002; 100:517-23.

[6] Cailhier JF, Partolina M, Vuthoori S, Wu S, Ko K, Watson S, Savill J, Hughes J, Lang RA. Conditional macrophage ablation demonstrates that resident macrophages initiate acute peritoneal inflammation. *J. Immunol.* 2005; 174:2336-42.

[7] Broche F, Tellado JM. Defense mechanisms of the peritoneal cavity. *Curr. Opin. Crit Care* 2001; 7:105-16.

[8] van Till JWO, van Veen SQ, van Ruler O, Lamme B, Gouma DJ, Boermeester MA. The innate immune response to secondary peritonitis. *Shock* 2007; 28:504-17.

[9] Ulloa L, Tracey KJ. The "cytokine profile": a code for sepsis. Trends Mol Biol 2005; 11:56-63.

[10] Hoesel LM, Ward PA. Mechanisms of inflammatory response syndrome in sepsis. *Drug Discov Today* 2004; 1:345-50.

[11] Opal SM. The host response to endotoxin, antilipopolysaccharide strategies, and the management of severe sepsis. *Int. J. Med. Microbiol.* 2007; 297:365-77.

[12] Surbatovic M, Radakovic S, Jovanovic K, Romic P. New strategies in multiple organ dysfunction syndrome for sepsis. *Srp. Arh Celok Lek* 2005; 133:379-83.

[13] Lucas S. The autopsy pathology of sepsis-related death. *Curr. Diagn Pathol.* 2007; 13:375-88.

[14] Lin E, Calvano SE, Lowry SF. Inflammatory cytokines and cell response in surgery. *Surgery* 2000; 127:117-26.

[15] Delogu G, Moretti S, Antonucci A. et al. Apoptosis and Surgical Trauma. Dysregulated Expression of Death and Survival Factors on Peripheral Lymphocytes. *Arch. Surg.* 2000; 135:1141-47.

[16] Liese AM, Siddiqi MQ, Siegel JH. et al. Augmented TNF-α and IL-10 production by primed human monocytes following interaction with oxidatively modified autologous erythrocytes. *J. Leukoc. Biol.* 2001; 70:289-96.

[17] dos Santos CC, Zhang H, Slutsky AS. From bench to bedside: bacterial growth and cytokines. *Crit. Care* 2002; 6:4-6.

[18] Meduri GU. Clinical review: A paradigm shift: the bidirectional effect of inflammation on bacterial growth. Clinical implications for patients with acute respiratory distress syndrome. *Crit. Care* 2002; 6:24-9.

[19] de Werra I, Zanetti G, Calandra T. et al. CD14 expression on monocytes and TNF-α production in patients with septic shock, cardiogenic shock or bacterial pneumonia. *Swiss Med Wkly* 2001; 131:35-40.

[20] Tjardes T, Neugebauer E. Sepsis research in the next millennium: concentrate on the software rather than the hardware. *Shock* 2002; 17:1-8.

[21] Jean-Baptiste E. Cellular mechanism in sepsis. *J. Intensive Care Med.* 2007; 22:63-72.

[22] Sorensen TI, Nielsen GG, Andersen PK, et al: Genetic and environmental influences on premature death in adult adoptees. *N. Engl. J. Med.* 1988; 318:727-32.

[23] Read RC, Teare DM, Pridmore AC, et al: The tumor necrosis factor polymorphism TNF (-308) is associated with susceptibility to meningococcal sepsis, but not with lethality. *Crit. Care Med* 2009; 37:1237-43.

[24] De Maio A, Torres MB, Reeves RH: Genetic determinants influencing the response to injury, inflammation and sepsis. *Shock* 2005; 23:11-7.

[25] Surbatovic M, Grujic K, Cikota B, Jevtic M, Filipovic N, Romic P, Strelic N, Magic Z. Polymorphisms of genes encoding tumor necrosis factor-alpha, interleukin-10, cluster of differentiation-14 and interleukin-1ra in critically ill patients. *J. Crit. Care* 2010; 5:542.e1-8.

[26] Gordon AC, Lagan AL, Aganna E, et al: TNF and TNFR polymorphisms in severe sepsis and septic shock: a prospective multicenter study. *Genes Immun*. 5:631-640, 2004.

[27] Mira JP, Cariou A, Grall F, et al: Association of TNF2, TNF-α Promoter Polymorphism, With Septic Shock Susceptibility and Mortality. A Multicenter Study. *JAMA* 282:561-568, 1999.

[28] O'Keefe GE, Hybki DL, Munford RS: The G → A single nucleotide polymorphism at the -308 position in the tumor necrosis factor alpha promoter increases the risk for severe sepsis after trauma. *J. Trauma* 52:817-825, 2002.

[29] Watanabe E, Hirasawa H, Oda S, et al: Extremely high interleukin-6 blood levels and outcome in the critically ill are associated with tumor necrosis factor- and interleukin-1-related gene polymorphisms. *Crit. Care Med.* 33:89-97, 2005.

[30] Tang GJ, Huang SL, Yien HW, et al: Tumor necrosis factor gene polymorphism and septic shock in surgical infection. *Crit. Care Med* 28:2733-2736, 2000.

[31] Barber RC, Aragaki CC, Rivera-Chavez FA, et al: TLR4 and TNF-α polymorphisms are associated with an increased risk for severe sepsis following burn injury. *J. Med. Genet* 41:808-813, 2004.

[32] Reid CL, Perrey C, Pravica V, et al: Genetic variation in proinflammatory and anti-inflammatory cytokine production in multiple organ dysfunction syndrome. *Crit. Care Med*. 30:2216-2221, 2002.

[33] Dianliang Z, Lieshou L, Zhiwei J, et al: Association of Plasma Levels of Tumor Necrosis Factor (TNF)-α and Its Soluble Receptors, Two Polymorphisms of the TNF Gene with Acute Severe Pancreatitis and Early Septic Shock Due to It. *Pancreas* 26:339-343, 2003.

[34] Powell JJ, Fearon KC, Siriwardena AK, et al: Evidence against a role for polymorphisms at tumor necrosis factor, interleukin-1 and interleukin-1-receptor antagonist gene loci in the regulation of disease severity in acute pancreatitis. *Surgery* 129:633-640, 2001.

[35] Waterer GW, Wunderink RG: Science review: Genetic variability in the systemic inflammatory response. *Crit. Care* 7:308-314, 2003.

[36] Papachristou GI, Clermont G, Sharma A, et al: Risk and Markers of Severe Acute Pancreatitis. *Gastroenterol. Clin. N. Am*. 36:277-296, 2007.

[37] Zhang DL, Zheng HM, Yu BJ, et al: Association of polymorphisms of IL and CD14 genes with acute severe pancreatitis and septic shock. *World J. Gastroenterol.* 11:4409-4413, 2005.

[38] Sabelnikovs O, Nikitina-Zake L, Zhuravlova J, et al: Association of IL-10 promoter polymorphism -1082 G/A with adverse outcome in severe sepsis and septic shock. *Crit. Care* 13(Suppl.1):P355, 2009 (abstr).

[39] Stanilova SA, Miteva LD, Karakolev ZT, et al: Interleukin-10-1082 promoter polymorphism in association with cytokine production and sepsis susceptibility. *Intensive Care Med.* 32:260-266, 2006.

[40] Schaaf BM, Boehmke F, Esnaashari H, et al: Pneumococcal Septic Shock Is Associated with the Interleukin-10-1082 Gene Promoter Polymorphism. *Am. J. Respir. Crit. Care Med.* 168:476-480, 2003.

[41] Shu Q, Fang X, Chen Q, et al: IL-10 polymorphism is associated with increased incidence of severe sepsis. *Chin. Med. J.* 116:1756-1759, 2003.

[42] Gong MN, Thompson BT, Williams PL, et al: Interleukin-10 polymorphism in position - 1082 and acute respiratory distress syndrome. *Eur. Respir. J.* 27:674-681, 2006.

[43] Sutherland AM, Walley KR, Russell JA: Polymorphisms in CD14, mannose-binding lectin, and Toll-like receptor 2 are associated with increased prevalence of infection in critically ill adults. *Crit Care Med.* 33:638-644, 2005.

[44] Yuan FF, Marks K, Wong M, et al: Clinical relevance of TLR2, TLR4, CD14 and FcγRIIA gene polymorphisms in Streptococcus pneumoniae infection. *Immunol. Cell Biol.* 86:268-270, 2008.

[45] Agnese DM, Calvano JE, Hahm SJ, et al: Human toll-like receptor 4 mutations but not CD14 polymorphisms are associated with an increased risk of gram-negative infections. *J. Infect Dis.* 186:1522-1525, 2002.

[46] Hubacek JA, Stuber F, Frohlich D, et al: The common functional C(-159)T polymorphism within the promoter region of the lipopolysaccharide receptor CD14 is not associated with sepsis development or mortality. *Genes Immun* 1:405-407, 2000.

[47] Nakada T, Hirasawa H, Oda S, et al: Influence of toll-like receptor 4, CD14, tumor necrosis factor and interleukin-10 gene polymorphisms on clinical outcome in Japanese critically Ill patients. *J. Surg. Res.* 129:322-328, 2005.

[48] Gibot S, Cariou A, Drouet L, et al: Association between a genomic polymorphism within the CD14 locus and septic shock susceptibility and mortality rate. *Crit. Care Med.* 30:969-973, 2002.

[49] Gu W, Dong H, Jiang DP, et al: Functional significance of CD14 promoter polymorphisms and their clinical relevance in a Chinese Han population. *Crit. Care Med.* 36:2274-2280, 2008.

[50] Fang XM, Schroder S, Hoeft A, et al: Comparison of two polymorphisms of the interleukin-1 gene family: Interleukin-1 receptor antagonist

polymorphism contributes to susceptibility to severe sepsis. *Crit. Care Med.* 27:1330-1334, 1999.

[51] Witkin SS, Gerber S, Ledger J: Influence of Interleukin-1 Receptor Antagonist Gene Polymorphism on Disease. *CID* 34:204-209, 2002.

[52] Arnalich F, Lopez-Maderuelo D, Codoceo R, et al: Interleukin-1 receptor antagonist gene polymorphism and mortality in patients with severe sepsis. *Clin. Exp. Immunol.* 127:331-336, 2002.

[53] Ma P, Chen D, Pan J, et al: Genomic polymorphism within interleukin-1 family cytokines influences the outcome of septic patients. *Crit. Care Med.* 30:1046-1050, 2002.

[54] Tumangger H, Jamil KF. Contribution of genes polymorphism to susceptibility and outcome of sepsis. T*he Egyptian Journal of Medical Human Genetics* 2010; 11: 97-103.

[55] Boontham P, Chandran P, Rowlands B, Eremin O. Surgical sepsis: dysregulation of immune function and therapeutic implications. *Surg. J. R. Coll Surg. Edinb. Irel.* 2003; 1:187-206.

[56] Hranjec T, Swenson BR, Dossett LA, Metzger R, Flohr TR, Popovsky KA, Bonatti HJ, May AK. Diagnosis-dependent relationships between cytokine levels and survival in patients admitted for surgical critical care. *J. Am. Coll Surg.* 2010; 210:833-846.

[57] Surbatovic M. Filipovic N, Radakovic S, Stankovic N, Slavkovic Z. Immune cytokine response in combat casualties: Blast or explosive trauma with or without secondary sepsis. *Mil. Med.* 2007; 172: 190-5.

[58] Dimopoulou I, Orfanos S, Kotanidou A, Livaditi O, et al. Plasma pro- and anti-inflammatory cytokine levels and outcome prediction in unselected critically ill patients. *Cytokine* 2008; 41:263-7.

[59] Volman TJH, Goris RJA, van der Meer JWM, Hendriks T. Tissue- and time-dependent upregulation of cytokine mRNA in a murine model for the multiple organ dysfunction syndrome. *Ann. Surg.* 2004; 240:142-50.

[60] Marshall JC. Principles of source control in the early management of sepsis. *Curr. Infect. Dis. Rep.* 2010; 12:345-353.

[61] Zugel N, Siebeck M, Geisler B, Lichtwark-Aschoff M, Gippner-Steppert C, Witte J, Jochum M. Circulating mediators and organ function in patients undergoing planned relaparotomy vs. conventional surgical therapy in severe secondary peritonitis. *Arch. Surg.* 2002; 137:590-9.

[62] Pflanz S, Timans JC, Cheung J, Rosales R, Kanzler H, Glibert J et al. IL-27, a heterodimeric cytokine composed of EBI3 and p28 protein, induces proliferation of naive CD4(+) T cells. *Immunity* 2002; 16:779-90.

[63] Wirtz S, Tubbe I, Galle PR, Schild HJ, Birkenbach M, Blumberg RS, Neurath MF. Protection from lethal septic peritonitis by neutralizing the biological function of interleukin 27. *JEM* 2006; 203:1875-81.

[64] Buyne OR, Bleichrodt RP, van Goor H, Verweij PE, Hendriks T. Plasminogen activator, but not systemic antibiotic therapy, prevents abscess formation in an experimental model of secondary peritonitis. *Br. J. Surg.* 2008; 95:1287-93.

[65] Hendriks T, Bleichrodt RP, Lome R, De Man BM, van Goor H, Buyne OR. Peritoneal cytokines predict mortality after surgical treatment of secondary peritonitis in the rat. *J. Am. Coll Surg.* 2010; 211:263-70.

[66] Jansson K, Redler B, Truedsson L, Magnuson A, Matthiessen P, Andersson M, Norgren L. Intraperitoneal cytokine response after major surgery: higher postoperative intraperitoneal versus systemic cytokine levels suggest the gastrointestinal tract as the major source of the postoperative inflammatory reaction. *Am. J. Surg.* 2004; 187:372-77.

[67] Osterberg J, Ljungdahl M, Lundholm M, Engstrand L, Haglund U. Microbial translocation and inflammatory response in patients with acute peritonitis. *Scand. J. Gastroenterol.* 2004; 39:657-64.

[68] Mulier S, Penninckx F, Verwaest C, Filez L, Aerts R, Fieuws S, Lauwers P. Factors affecting mortality in generalized postoperative peritonitis: multivariate analysis in 96 patients. *World J. Surg.* 2003; 27:379-84.

In: Liver Disease and Peritonitis
Editor: Mao Kang Voung et al. ISBN 978-1-61942-080-9

Chapter 2

Pediatric Non-Alcoholic Fatty Liver Disease

***Vincent Biank*[1] *and Ramin Alemzadeh*[*2]**

Department of Pediatrics, Division of Gastroenterology, Medical College of Wisconsin, Milwaukee, WI[1], US

Department of Pediatrics, Division of Endocrinology and Diabetes, University of Illinois at Chicago, Chicago, IL, US[2]

Abstract

Non-alcoholic fatty liver disease (NAFLD) is the metabolic consequence of obesity and metabolic syndrome. The incidence of childhood NAFLD has significantly increased in relation to the increasing prevalence of childhood obesity and its metabolic sequelae: dyslipidemia, hypertension and type 2 diabetes mellitus. As the incidence of childhood NAFLD has increased, so too has the more severe histologic form of NAFLD known as non-alcoholic steatohepatitis (NASH). NASH, which is characterized by inflammation, ballooning degeneration, and fibrosis, may progress to chronic, irreversible liver disease or even cirrhosis during childhood. Based on current trends, NAFLD and consequently

[*]Correspondence: Ramin Alemzadeh, MD, Professor of Pediatrics, Chief, Division of Endocrinology & Diabetes, Department of Pediatrics, M/C 856, University of Illinois at Chicago, 840 S. Wood Street, Chicago, IL 60612, Tel: 312-996-1795, Fax: 312-996-8218, Email: ralemzad@uic.edu

NASH are expected to become the most common causes of end-stage liver disease in both children and young adults, especially among male subjects. While the precise underlying pathophysiologic mechanism for development of NAFLD has not been identified, excessive fatty acid availability contributes to steatosis and the metabolic abnormalities associated with NAFLD. Indeed, increased adipocyte insulin resistance and lipolytic activity with marked elevation of circulating fatty acids are the likely pathogenic mechanisms leading to hepatic steatosis and, consequently, NAFLD. However, the factors influencing an individual's susceptibility for the development and progression of liver disease, such as NASH or cirrhosis, remain elusive. In addition, significant ethnic and gender differences association with the pediatric metabolic syndrome and NAFLD remain unexplained. Therefore, effective strategies are needed for identifying and treating NAFLD and preventing the progression to NASH and end stage liver disease.

Keywords: Obesity, fatty liver disease, insulin resistance, cirrhosis

Introduction

In the late 1970's chronic liver disease associated with obesity was described as a new and separate clinical entity.[1, 2] Eventually, the term NAFLD was developed to encompass a wide spectrum of disease states ranging from simple benign hepatic steatosis to NASH. NAFLD may be further classified into either primary, associated with obesity and insulin resistance, or secondary, resulting from various genetic, metabolic, or infectious causes or from a variety of medications/toxins.[3] NASH, on the other hand, is a subtype of NAFLD and remains a patho-clinical entity characterized by the development of histological changes of inflammation and fibrosis in the liver associated with excess fat deposition that are nearly identical to those induced by excessive alcohol intake, but in the absence of alcohol abuse.[4]

In children, primary NAFLD has reached epidemic proportions and is the leading cause of unexplained elevation in liver transaminases and the most common chronic liver disease in the Western World.[4] In the United States, the prevalence rates for NAFLD and NASH have increased from previous estimates and now range from 17% to 33% for NAFLD and 5.7% to 17% for NASH.[5] Paralleling the increasing prevalence of obesity and type 2 diabetes in the pediatric population, NAFLD and consequently NASH is expected to become one of the most common causes of end-stage liver disease in both children and young adults.[6] In this section, we will discuss the prevalence and pathophysiology of NAFLD, as well as explore some the risk factors for developing NAFLD and subsequently NASH including potential genetic links. We will also discuss the natural history, and diagnosis of NAFLD in the pediatric population as well as touch on some of the controversies in managing what is expected to become the leading cause of end-stage liver disease in both children and adults.

Prevalence of NAFLD

NAFLD is the most common cause of chronic liver disease in children and adolescents in the western hemisphere.[7] Schwimmer et al reported that 9.6% of the American population aged 2 to 19 years have NAFLD based on autopsy findings.[7] However, the prevalence of NAFLD has been reported as high as 38% among obese subjects,[7] with similar prevalence rates ranging from 24% to 53% in European and Asian populations.[8-11] Despite these alarming results there are several inherent challenges in estimating the prevalence of NAFLD. The first is making the diagnosis. At present, NAFLD and NASH are defined as a patho-clinical entity characterized by the development of histological changes of inflammation and fibrosis in the liver associated with excess fat deposition. As such, the inherent challenge is that, currently, the only definitive means of making the diagnosis is via liver biopsy.[4, 12, 13] Although alternative clinical diagnostic definitions have been utilized to avoid the invasive nature of liver biopsy such as the presence of persistently unexplained elevated ALT, these definitions have yet to be validated.[3] Alternatively, several imaging modalities have also been developed to estimate or quantify the amount of fatty infiltrate within the liver parenchyma ranging from simple ultrasound to MRI spectroscopy. These imaging modalities fail to identify the degree of inflammation and hepatocyte injury associate with this chronic inflammatory condition.[3] Fibroscan is a noninvasive imaging device which can be used to estimate the degree of fibrosis within the liver, but has not been standardized in children. As a result, despite these technological advancements, liver biopsy remains the only definite means of diagnosing NAFLD and consequently NASH.

Another inherent challenge in determining the prevalence of NAFLD and consequently NASH is defining the population to investigate. It is well known that NAFLD is associated with insulin resistance and obesity.[14] As such the current estimated prevalence of NAFLD is estimated to be around 20-30% for obese adolescents,[3, 15] however, if we examine the general population the prevalence of NASH is only 5-7%.[3, 15] Therefore, the population one chooses to examine dramatically impacts the prevalence of the disease. More concerning, however, is that despite the population one chooses to examine, the prevalence of NAFLD and NASH appears to be increasing especially among adolescent males such that reports now documenting that almost 50% of obese males have NAFLD.[15] The rise in NAFLD and NASH prevalence has paralleled the increasing prevalence of obesity among children and adolescents aged 2-19 years of age, with 12% at or above the 97th percentile and over 30% at or above the 85% percentile for BMI for age according to the most recent NHANES data.[16]

Pathophysiology of NAFLD

Since 2001, Sanyal and Marchesini documented that NASH is associated with both peripheral[17] and hepatic[18] insulin resistance by using a hyperinsulinemic euglycemic clamp, the gold-standard for assessing insulin sensitivity in vivo. This conclusion was further strengthened by additional data showing that being overweight and/or obesity could lead to inflammatory hepatic injury[19] and fibrosis,[20] with insulin resistance being an independent predictive factor. These findings eventually lead to the "double hit" hypothesis of disease pathogenesis with the first 'hit' represented by fatty infiltration of the liver commonly associated with obesity.[21] However, increase in fat deposition alone is insufficient in explaining the inflammation or fibrosis associated with NASH, thus, oxidative stress, due to excessive production of reactive oxygen species (ROS) within the cells has been implicated as a possible factor responsible for the second "hit" leading to steatohepatitis. Over the last decade, however, new findings have all but abandoned this simple theory to suggest that NAFLD and subsequently NASH is a multi-factorial process resulting from the interactions of several organ systems and an individual's dietary intake which ultimately leads from over nutrition to insulin resistance, resulting in liver steatatosis, and finally, to inflammation and fibrosis.

To start, over nutrition is the result of a complex interaction of one's genetic make-up and environmental triggers with central appetite regulation, food intake, energy expenditure and metabolic regulation all influencing the overall result. Specifically, over 100 genes have been identified to be in association with obesity but less than a handful account of more than even a small percentage of the severely obese population. This fact suggests that an individual's genetic make-up may play only a small role in their risk of becoming obese. Regardless of the cause, consumption of excess calories consistently results in the development of obesity, and consequently, the comorbidities associated with it. Obesity has several unintended consequences which ultimately affects the development of NAFLD via a common pathway of lipotoxicity leading to hepatocellular injury, inflammation, and fibrosis. First there is the adipose tissue itself. Numerous studies have identified that increased visceral adipose tissue is strongly correlated with the development of NASH.[14, 22-24] One proposed mechanism is that increased visceral adipose tissue results in dysregulation of visceral lipolysis with a subsequent increase in free fatty acid production. Sedentary activity which is both a consequence and a predisposing factor associated with obesity also leads to increased free fatty acid production as a result of insulin resistance and decreased beta oxidation in muscles. Finally, the increased dietary fat intake associated with obesity results in additional free fatty acids such that together these three factors account for close to three-fourths of the lipid accumulation in the liver. It is this accumulation of fat which ultimately leads to the production of numerous inflammatory cytokine including tumor necrosis factor (TNF)-α, interleukin (IL)-6 and monocyte chemo-attractant protein-1 all of which play important roles in the promotion of liver injury and fibrosis. Park and colleagues recently demonstrated that two of these cytokines, IL-6 and TNF-α, play a central role in the promotion of liver inflammation and tumor-genesis in dietary and genetic obesity.[25] In addition, IL-6 serum levels are elevated in obese patients and decrease proportionately when weight loss occurs[26, 27]. In addition, enhanced TNF-α expression in adipose tissue of obese subjects also decreases following weight loss.[28] This data in conjunction with mouse models of NASH clearly demonstrate the toxicity of excess lipid accumulation.

Demographics, Genetic Predispositions and Risk Factors for NAFLD

NAFLD may affect any age or ethnic group. Adult studies frequently support a female preponderance NAFLD,[2, 29] however, in children, males are more frequently affected with male to female ratios reported as high as 2:1 in epidemiologic studies.[30-32] This switch from an increased male to female prevalence suggests sex hormones may be associated with the development of NAFLD.[33] Furthermore most children are diagnosed between 11.5 and 13.5 years of age at the peak of pubertal insulin resistance again, implying a role for sex hormones in the development of NAFLD.[34] In children and teens, the prevalence of NAFLD seems to be different among different ethnic groups, with the highest prevalence among Hispanic people and the lowest among African American children.[7] It has been suggested that differences in body fat distribution and body composition among the various ethnic groups may explain these differences in NAFLD prevalence. For instance, Hispanic individuals have a higher proportion of body fat and higher waist to hip ratio than their taller counterparts.[35]

Although over 100 genes have been associated with obesity, each mutation only accounts for a small fraction of the risk for becoming obese. These findings suggest that obesity is a polygenetic disease which likely results from the interaction of several polymorphisms in conjunction with the proper environmental triggers. A similar conclusion can be made for both NAFLD and NASH. Both environmental and genetic factors have been suggested to explain the presence of NASH. In analogy to the proposed mechanisms of damage associated with alcoholic liver disease, oxidative stress, due to excessive production of reactive oxygen species (ROS) within the cells, has been indicated as a possible factor responsible for steatohepatitis. Based on this hypothesis, several candidate genes have been investigated and identified as increasing susceptibility to development of adult onset NASH including the microsomal triglyceride transfer protein (MTP) which regulates the incorporation of triglycerides into apolipoprotein B and a key enzyme for the assembly and secretion of VLDL from hepatocytes,[36, 37] the manganese superoxide dismutase (MnSOD) gene which catalyzes the conversion of two molecules of superoxide anion, a highly unstable ROS, into hydrogen peroxide and oxygen more stable ROS,[36, 38] and Phosphatidylethanolamine *N*-methyltransferase (PEMT) which is required for hepatic secretion of triacylglycerol in very low density lipoproteins (VLDL).[39, 40] More recently, polymorphisms of TNF-α have been recognized in association with adult onset NASH suggesting that the interaction of cytokines with oxidative stress and lipid peroxidation may play a key role in the progression from simple steatosis to steatohepatitis and ultimately fibrosis.[38, 41] In addition to these individual candidate gene investigations, a genome-wide association study conducted in 2008 on adults identified a polymorphism in the patatin-like phosphate family of genes that was associated with a 2 fold increase in hepatic fat content for homozygous individuals compared to non-carriers. Despite the increase risk associated with the numerous genetic mutations, no single mutation accounts for a significant fraction of the NASH population.

From a clinical perspective, visceral obesity and the presence of insulin resistance appear to have the greatest correlation with NASH. This has been documented in several adult studies, but only insulin resistance appears to have a similar correlation in children[42]. Visceral obesity is usually associated with impaired insulin activity, overflow of portal triglycerides and overproduction of inflammatory cytokines.[43] Even though many surrogate parameters have been proposed as markers of visceral adiposity, waist circumference remains the simplest and most widely used.[44] Additional clinical risk factors to consider would include the presence of acanthosis nigrans which is a darkening and/or thickening of the skin around the neck and extensor surfaces of the extremities and digits. Acanthosis nigrans is believed to be a surrogate marker for insulin resistance and therefore is frequently correlated with the presence of NAFLD/NASH.

Several laboratory markers have also been identified as indirect markers of NAFLD. Fierbinteanu-Braticevicil documented significant differences in the amount of malondialdehyde and serum gluthation in patients with NASH compared to controls. Both of these markers are the result of increased reactive oxidative stress and mitochondrial DNA damage in association with activated cellular lipid peroxidation. More common clinically, C- reactive protein has frequently been identified as an independent predictive factor of NASH.[44-46]

Natural History and Metabolic and Nutritional Profile of NAFLD

Development of NAFLD, NASH and End Stage Liver Disease

The spectrum of liver injury in NAFLD consists of several distinct stages ranging from "benign" hepatic steatosis to steatohepatitis (NASH) to advanced fibrosis and cirrhosis (Figure 1).[47, 48].

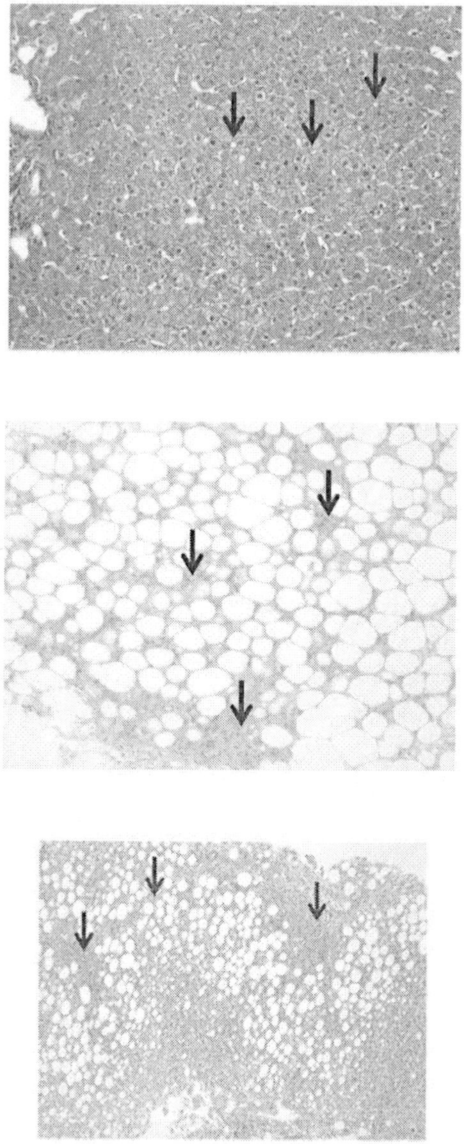

Figure 1. Histopathology of NAFLD and NASH. (a) Hematoxylin and Eosin (HandE) stain of NAFLD demonstrating mild increase in hepatic steatosis as identified by the arrows. (b) HandE stain of NASH with markedly increased hepatic steatosis and evidence of hepatitis as identified by the arrows. (c) Trichrome stain of NASH with markedly increased hepatic steatosis and evidence of fibrosis as identified by the arrows.

Hepatic steatosis is the most common presentation, is readily reversible, and does not progress to either fibrosis or steatohepatitis in the majority of patients.[2, 29, 49] Indeed, the rate of progression of NAFLD is believed to be related to its histologic severity.[50] On the other hand, insulin resistance is a common finding in pediatric NAFLD.

Therefore, some of the clinical features associated with insulin resistance and metabolic syndrome such as obesity, type 2 diabetes mellitus, and dyslipidemia are common co-morbidities in children and adolescents with NAFLD.[3, 42, 51, 52] In fact, it has been shown that the presence of metabolic syndrome is associated with progression of NAFLD to NASH and liver fibrosis.[53] Consequently, there is significant controversy about the clinical significance and prognosis of "bland" steatosis such that the benign nature of simple steatosis has been disputed. In several adult studies, morbidly obese patients have required liver transplantation following either proximal gastric or jejunoileal bypass.[54-56] However, data on the prognosis of NAFLD in children remains rather limited.

Some studies have reported cases of cirrhosis occurring in young children,[57] while other studies have reported cases of children with NAFLD who do not develop cirrhosis until adulthood.[58, 59] Several studies evaluating alterations in fibrosis stage have demonstrated that while fibrosis may remain stable or even improved spontaneously in some individuals,[12, 60-63] it has a tendency to progress overtime.[12, 60-62] Central obesity and features of metabolic syndrome, especially elevated triglycerides with low HLD cholesterol levels increase the risk of hepatic fibrosis and consequently progression of disease.[50] Together this variability in prognosis suggests the presence of fibrosis may indicate irreversible hepatic injury.[64] In fact, Feldstein et al reported that children with NAFLD seen in a tertiary care center may be associated with a significantly shorter survival compared to the general population and that children with NAFLD may develop end stage liver disease requiring liver transplantation.[65]

More advanced stages of NAFLD appear to be associated with older age, higher body adiposity, diabetes, hypertension, elevated triglycerides, and/or insulin resistance.[50] In addition, an AST/ALT ratio > 1 may also suggest more severe disease in adults.[64, 66] However, review of the various pediatric NAFLD fails to identify which factors are independently associated with elevated liver enzymes.[50] Alternatively, the progression of liver fibrosis is accompanied by significant improvement or resolution of other features of NAFLD, including steatosis, inflammation and ballooning of hepatocyte.[12] Therefore, the severity of hepatic fibrosis may be the only practical histologic feature for predicting the long-term outcomes of pediatric patients with NAFLD. In addition, it is likely that the long-term complications of NAFLD might have been undocumented since the characteristic features of macrovesicular steatosis may not be apparent in the late stages of disease, leading to a picture of "bland" or "cryptogenic" cirrhosis rather than NAFLD-related cirrhosis.[50]

Matteoni *et al* retrospectively compared clinical characteristics and outcomes of 98 adult patients with different types of NAFLD over an average follow-up period of 8.3 years.[67] They demonstrated that the outcome of cirrhosis and liver-related death was not uniform across the spectrum of NAFLD. Furthermore, they demonstrated that poor outcomes were more common in individuals with advanced types of NAFLD (Types 3 and 4), designated as NASH.[67] This study suggests that histological findings may have prognostic value in patients with NAFLD, while other tertiary care center studies have documented progression of histologic NASH to cirrhosis and hepatocellular carcinoma. These studies are limited by their small patient samples and/or short duration of follow-up.[47, 68-70] Rafiq *et al*, recently observed that liver-related mortality of an adult NASH cohort was 17.5% in comparison to only 2.7% for the non-NASH group over a median 18.5 year follow-up period,[71] thus confirming higher liver-related mortality rates among NASH patients compared to non-NASH patients during a long follow-up periods.[49, 70, 71]

While NAFLD is very common in the pediatric population, there have been few long-term studies evaluating the long-term prognosis of NAFLD in children. Since large number of children are affected by NAFLD, it is critical to establish a better understanding of the natural history of pediatric fatty liver and its progression.[7] Although some studies have observed cases of cirrhotic stage disease in children[7, 57] or cases of children with NAFLD with progression to cirrhosis in young adulthood,[58, 59] cirrhosis is not considered to be a natural consequence of pediatric NASH. Baldridge et al suggested that the delay in presentation of cirrhosis until adulthood may be due to the short duration of the process or the introduction of a cofactor after childhood.[72] For instance, cirrhosis has been observed in some patients with NAFLD associated with hypopituitarism and bronchopulmonary syndrome,[65, 72-75] which adversely affect long-term prognosis in this patient population despite optimal treatment of endocrine disorders. In contrast, hepatic fibrosis is frequently observed in pediatric NASH. Kinugasa *et al* observed elevation of serum transaminases among 12% of obese children and documented hepatic fibrosis in one-third of children with elevated liver enzymes who underwent liver biopsies.[57]

In a study involving a group of 24 predominantly obese children, large-droplet steatosis was observed in all patients; and fibrosis was observed in 17% to 71% with varying degrees of severity.[76] In seven patients, fibrosis was moderately severe, while an additional patient had evidence of cirrhosis. Schwimmer et al found that simple steatosis was present in 16% of subjects, and advanced fibrosis in 8% of 100 children with clinical features of NAFLD.[15] On the other hand, a study involving 84 obese and overweight children with clinical diagnosis of NAFLD and elevated transaminases confirmed by liver biopsy observed that 58% of patients had mild fibrosis, whereas 37.3% and 4.7% of patients had moderate and severe fibrosis, respectively.[51] Recently, a longitudinal study evaluating the long-term follow-up of children with NAFLD for up to 20 years, showed that NAFLD is a disease of progressive potential.[65] While some children presented with cirrhosis, others progressed with advanced fibrosis or cirrhosis during follow-up and some developed end-stage liver disease required liver transplantation. In this series, children with NAFLD had significantly shorter long-term survival as compared to survival rate in the age- and gender-matched children in the general population. Also, children with NAFLD had a 13.8-fold higher mortality risk or requiring liver transplantation than age- and gender-matched children.

Pattern types of steatohepatitis have been found to be influenced by age, gender, race, ethnicity, and severity of obesity.[15] While older age has been found to be independently associated with increased liver fibrosis in some series,[51] other investigators have found that children with advanced stages of fibrosis tended to be younger than those with lesser degrees of fibrosis[77] suggesting that potential unidentified susceptibility genes predispose to the more aggressive course in these children. Furthermore, males appear to be more commonly affected than females according to a number of studies.[76, 78, 79] Schwimmer *et al* observed that girls with moderate (type 2) NASH were more likely to be prepubertal (Tanner 1) with similar hormonal profile compared to young boys with type 2 NASH.[15] However, girls with mild (type 1) NASH were more likely to be late stages of puberty (Tanner 4) with higher estrogen levels suggesting that sex hormones may be possible mediators in the development of NASH or even play protective roles.

Alternatively, plasma insulin levels increase with corresponding decrease in insulin sensitivity during puberty.[80, 81] In a group of prepubertal and pubertal children, pubertal maturation was accompanied by a 32% reduction in insulin sensitivity with similar changes across gender, ethnicity, and obesity.[82] Thus, sex steroid hormones and insulin resistance associated with pubertal development may account for the significance of developmental stage in the onset of NAFLD.[77] Indeed, Patton *et al* observed that lower early stages of puberty were predictive of higher fibrosis scores, suggesting that hormonal changes associated with pubertal development may influence disease severity.[77] However, these authors were not able to determine whether children with mild fibrosis (zone 1) would progress into definite NASH and/or children with definite NASH regress to borderline zone 3 or simple steatosis.

Obesity and diabetes have been reported to be independent predictors of hepatic fibrosis in adults.[19, 83] While some studies observed an association between higher body mass index (BMI) and severity of fibrosis,[51, 52] clinical data from the NASH Clinical Research Network documented no association between BMI and severity of fibrosis.[3] However, it is likely that body fat distribution (visceral versus subcutaneous)[84] is a more important determinant of fibrosis than BMI. Furthermore, body fat distribution affects insulin sensitivity and varies by race and ethnicity and therefore may account for the differences in the prevalence between various ethnicities.[42] For instance, it has been shown that Hispanic children have significantly higher body fat and percentage fat than Caucasian and African American children.[85] Patton et al observed that Hispanic ethnicity was predictive of fibrosis severity when comparing those with mild and moderate degrees of fibrosis in a group of children with NAFLD.[3] In addition, metabolic syndrome and its individual components have been shown to be present in almost all children with biopsy-proven NAFLD.[42, 52, 77] Recently, it was shown that metabolic syndrome is common among children with NAFLD and is associated with severity of steatosis, hepatocellular ballooning, mean NAFLD activity score (NAS), NAFLD pattern, and the presence of advanced fibrosis.[86] Individual metabolic syndrome features, particularly central obesity and insulin resistance, were also associated with severity of NAFLD.

In recent years, the natural history of NAFLD has become better defined, since understanding of the disease process has become more refined due to the availability of long-term follow-up data. While simple steatosis is generally nonprogressive, a small percentage of patients with simple steatosis may progress to NASH with potential progression to cirrhosis.[65] Nevertheless, the morbidity and mortality data in children with NAFLD and NASH-related liver disease and progression to cirrhosis are limited due to scarcity of long-term studies.

Approach to Diagnosis of NAFLD

Clinical Presentation

The majority of children and adolescents with NAFLD and NASH are asymptomatic with mild, incidental elevation of aminotransferases during routine screening for obesity-related complications.[34, 87] Furthermore, no specific symptoms can differentiate NAFLD or NASH from other types of liver disease. The diagnosis of NAFLD requires the exclusion of other specific etiologies of liver disease (Figure 2). The majority of patients have one or more features of metabolic syndrome, including obesity, impaired glucose tolerance, dyslipidemia, hypertension, polycystic ovary syndrome and sleep apnea. Children may sometimes complain of fatigue and right upper quadrant abdominal discomfort or epigastric pain.

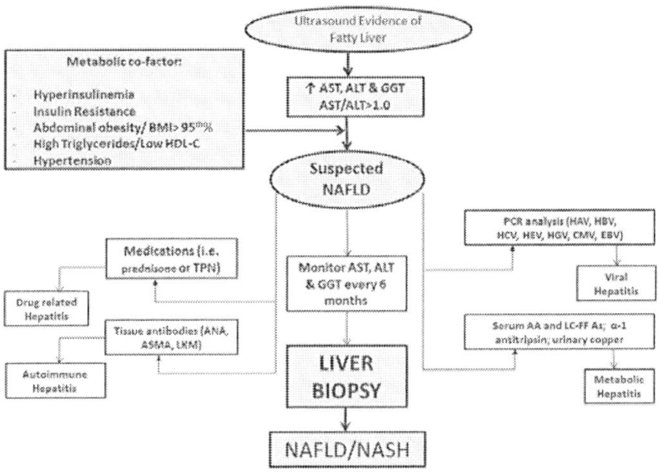

Figure 2. Diagnostic Algorithm for Suspected NAFLD. Algorithm adapted from Manco et al.[151] Abbreviations: Amino Acids (AA); Antinuclear Antibodies (ANA); Anti-Smooth Muscle Antibody (ASMA); Cytomegalovirus (CMV); Epstein Barr Virus (EBV); Hepatitis Viruses (HAV; HBV; HCV; HEV; HGV); Liver Kidney Microsomal antibodies (LKM); Long Chain Free Fatty Acids (LC-FFAs); Polymerase Chain Reaction; (PCR); Total Parenteral nutrition (TPN). Adapted from Manco et al. Nonalcoholic fatty liver disease in children. J Am Coll of Nut 2008; 27 (6): 667-676.

The children are often overweight or obese with central (abdominal) adiposity. Other physical signs of metabolic syndrome or insulin resistance include acanthosis nigrans which is present in approximately one third to one-half of children.[42, 76] In addition, mild hepatomegaly may be noted in 33% to 51% of children with NAFLD.[2, 88] Rarely, cutaneous stigmata of cirrhosis (spider angioma, jaundice, scleral icterus, palmar erythema and gynectomastia) may be present with features of portal hypertension (ascites, asterixis and encephalopathy) if the liver disease is advanced.

Diagnosis - Laboratory Evaluations

NAFLD should be suspected as a cause of asymptomatic moderate elevation of serum aminotransferases (less than 1.5 times the upper limit of normal).[89] However, it should be noted that NAFLD can be present with fluctuating or even normal AST and ALT.[90] The AST/ALT ratio is usually less than one, but this ratio increases as fibrosis progresses.[63] Nevertheless, similar to other types of liver disorders, an AST/ALT ratio greater than one may suggest advanced fibrosis. In a group of children with NAFLD, Patton et al showed a strong association between serum AST and histologic features of liver biopsies,[77] suggesting that evaluation of serum aminotransferases levels can be a useful screening tool for pediatric NAFLD in overweight children and adolescents.[91] Furthermore, serum gamma glutamyl transferase (GGT) has been found to be a useful diagnostic tool in NAFLD and a marker for metabolic syndrome.[92] Feldstein et al reported that serum GGT was elevated in 88% of patients[65] and almost one third of the patients met the conclusive diagnostic criteria for metabolic syndrome. Indeed, elevated serum GGT concentrations have been associated with several cardiovascular disease risk factors[93, 94] acting as a surrogate marker of oxidative stress and insulin resistance.[65] Also, serum adiponectin level is decreased in NAFLD and can predict the severity of liver disease.[66] While nonspecific autoantibodies against smooth muscle determinants, may be detected in somewhat low titers in up to 3% of adults with NAFLD, the prevalence in children is unknown.[95] Finally, it is critical that comprehensive evaluation is performed and other causes of liver such as viral hepatitis, α-1-antitrypsin deficiency, hemochromatosis, Wilson's disease, autoimmune hepatitis, fatty acid oxidation defects, lipodystrophy, and total parenteral nutrition are excluded. In adolescents, alcohol use must also be excluded as clinical causes of liver disease. Finally, drug-related liver injuries have been reported with a number of medications such as tetracycline, prednisone, amiodarone, valproic acid, statins, niacin and methotrexate.

Radiological Evaluation

Radiologic imaging techniques, including ultrasound, computed tomography (CT), magnetic resonance imaging, and magnetic resonance spectroscopy (MRS) may detect fatty infiltration of the liver. However, these imaging methods are limited since they cannot detect presence of liver inflammation and fibrosis.[96]

Ultrasound

Hepatic ultrasound (US) is a rather inexpensive, noninvasive technique, and widely used in clinical practice to detect hepatic fatty infiltration. Ultrasound may show liver steatosis as a hyperechogenic image, that is, "bright liver." However, in order to detect hepatic steatosis by sonography technique, hepatocyte fat content should exceed 15% to 30%.[97] In addition, ultrasonography may be technically difficult to perform in patients with significant central obesity since it has been shown that ultrasound has limited accuracy likely due to technical problems in performing ultrasound in such patients.[98] Several studies have reported grading of hepatic fat content using ultrasound; however, this is rather subjective.[99, 100]

CT Scan

The use of unenhanced CT has been proposed as a tool for quantification of the degree of hepatic steatosis.[101] However, others reported that the use of unenhanced CT did not quantify macrovesicular steatosis less than 30%, which made this technique clinically limited as a reliable diagnostic tool.[102] In addition, CT scanning has the disadvantage of exposing subjects to ionizing radiation.

Magnetic Resonance Imaging

Magnetic resonance imaging (MRI) is highly sensitive for quantification of hepatic steatosis and is considered a superior technique compared to US and CT scan.[100, 103] While the cost of MRI is significantly higher than US, it is a more desirable study in that it detects minor changes in hepatic fat content in

NAFLD and NASH and it is not influenced by severity of hepatic fibrosis.[100] Indeed, Fishbein et al showed the fast-MRI was a very sensitive method in detecting low levels (< 18%) of hepatic fat fraction (HFF) in obese children compared to serum ALT screening. Another study showed that only 48% of obese children with intrahepatic fat accumulation (as evidenced by HFF ≥ 5.5% using fast-MRI) had abnormal ALT levels.[30] Pacifico et al showed that obese children with elevated ALT had a much higher mean level of MRI HFF than obese children with normal serum ALT.[104] They also observed that US was rather limited in grading steatosis compared with quantitative assessment of HFF using fat-MRI.[104]

Magnetic Resonance Spectroscopy (MRS)

This noninvasive technique measures hepatic triglycerides quantitatively. It is considered safe and reproducible. However, further studies are needed to determine its effectiveness for stages of fibrosis in NAFLD.[105]

Fibrosan

Currently, fibroscan or transient elastography is a noninvasive technique for determination of hepatic fibrosis stiffness. Fibroscan is being assessed for evaluation of stages of fibrosis in NAFLD and NASH. Using fibroscan, Foucher et al observed that liver stiffness correlated with the severity of hepatic fibrosis in a group of patients with chronic liver disease, including chronic hepatitis B, C, and NASH.[106] However, the role of fibroscan role in obese NAFLD patients remains to be established.[107]

Histologic Evaluation

Histologic criteria for the diagnosis of NAFLD require 5% to 10% macrovesicular hepatic steatosis with or without other pathologic features such as fibrosis and inflammation. In general, 4 types of NAFLD histologic criteria have been described: (1) simple steatosis only; (2) simple steatosis and lobular inflammation; (3) steatosis and ballooning degeneration; and (4) steatosis and ballooning degeneration with either Mallory's hyaline or fibrosis.[108] Matteoni et al observed that while types 1 and 2 NAFLD typically follow a nonprogressive course, types 3 and 4 NAFLD tend to have a progressive course.[67] However, others have developed a scoring system which consists of 4 stages of NAFLD: (1) NASH described as steatosis in zone 3, occasional ballooning, and intra-acinar inflammation with pericellular fibrosis; (2) features of stage 1 plus sinusoidal and periportal fibrosis; (3) bridging fibrosis between zones 3 and 1; and (4) cirrhosis[13]

On the other hand The NAFLD Activity Score (NAS) developed by NASH Clinical Research Network provides a histologic scoring system for diagnosis of NAFLD.[109] The NAS evaluates 3 pathologic features: macrosteatosis in zone 3, inflammation, and hepatocyte ballooning. In addition, the inclusion of other histologic features such as Mallory's hyaline, perisinusoidal fibrosis, portal inflammation, acidophilic bodies, glycogenated nuclei, Kupffer cells and lipogranulomas are used in order to enhance the diagnostic criteria for NASH. Therefore, histologic activity is graded 0 to 8 and fibrosis, 0 to 4. NASH is confirmed with a score of 5 or greater.[109] However, NAS has not been used extensively in clinical practice to establish the diagnosis of NASH since this scoring system was developed for clinical trials of NASH. Further, histologic features of NASH differ in children compared to adults. In children, the histologic evaluation often reveals mononuclear inflammatory infiltrate that is periportal rather than perivenular. Mallory bodies are rarely present in pediatric NAFLD, and fibrosis has a periportal rather than pericellular distribution.[15, 110] Also, pathologic features of NASH in morbidly obese patients may show changes in the portal area rather than central areas of a liver biopsy, which may result in liver biopsy sampling error NAFLD. However, liver biopsy remains the gold standard for diagnosis of NASH.

Biomarkers

There are currently several noninvasive biomarkers which are being assessed for diagnosis of NASH by evaluating hepatic steatosis and fibrosis.[110] Indeed, three types of biomarkers are under assessment for clinical use which may replace liver biopsy. It has been shown that a pro-inflammatory state and oxidative stress and apoptosis play important roles in the pathogenesis of NAFLD.[111-114] It has been observed that elevated serum cytokeratin-18 (CK-18) and caspase-cleaved CK-18 in adult patients with NAFLD are highly sensitive and specific markers for diagnosis of NASH.[112, 113] Other biomarkers such as M30 and M65 antigens, adiponectin and resistin have also been suggested as reliable diagnostic tools for diagnosis of NASH.[114]

Using four predictors of NAFLD [BMI, waist circumference, triglycerides and gammaglutamyl transpeptidase (GGT)], Bedogni et al developed the fatty liver index (FLI) (reference range 0 to 100) for determination of hepatic steatosis[115] and confirmed by hepatic sonographic evaluation. They excluded steatosis in those with FLI<30, and confirmed steatosis in individuals with FLI>60.

FibroTest (FibroSure) and ActiTest are both noninvasive blood tests for estimation of degree of fibrosis which offer an alternative to liver biopsy.[116] These commercially available laboratory tests quantitate necroinflammatory activity and fibrosis along with 5 markers:

- a2-macroglobulin, apolipoprotein A1, haptoglobulin, total bilirubin, and GGT corrected
- for age and gender. The ActiTest includes the FibroTest plus ALT. However, the accuracy of both tests are questioned in individuals with acute hepatitis, cholestasis or with Gilbert's syndrome.

In addition, Poynard et al described the diagnostic value of another biomarker called SteatoTest for detection of steatosis or NASH.[117] This test uses FibroTest-ActiTest along with glucose, triglycerides, cholesterol and BMI adjusted to age and gender. While SteatoTest is used primarily for evaluation of steatosis, NashTest varies slightly in that it attempts to differentiate steatosis from NASH.[116] To date, there has been no extensive validation of these biomarkers in children and adolescents with NAFLD and/or NASH.

Management

Currently, there is no approved medical management for NAFLD. Children and adolescents with NAFLD are recommended to make lifestyle changes with targeted medical management of underlying insulin resistance, hypertension, dyslipidemias and obesity. On the other hand, medical interventions are utilized in the treatment of NASH since it poses a high risk of progression to hepatic cirrhosis.

Diet Lifestyle Modifications

The initial approach to the management of NAFLD consists of weight loss by implementing lifestyle changes with diet and exercise. Although there has been no controlled study evaluating the role of weight loss for treatment of NAFLD, weight reduction has been demonstrated to decrease body fat resulting in reduced insulin resistance. It has been shown that lifestyle intervention with diet and increased physical activity induces weight loss and is associated with a significant improvement in liver histology and laboratory abnormalities in pediatric NAFLD.[118] Indeed, aerobic exercise may prevent the development of steatosis since insulin sensitivity is enhanced through peripheral lipolysis, inhibiting lipid synthesis and facilitating fatty acid oxidation.[119] In adults, a target loss of 10% of the baseline weight has been suggested as the initial goal for a BMI greater than 25. The aimed is to reduce AST and ALT levels with attenuation of hepatomegaly.[120] On the other hand, Ueno et al evaluated the metabolic effects of restricted diet and exercise in a small group of adults with NAFLD.[121] While patients in the diet and exercise group had improvements in BMI, ALT and AST levels, total cholesterol, and decreased serum glucose with improvement in steatosis on liver biopsy compared with control group, there was no reduction in inflammation or fibrosis. Nevertheless, it has been shown that weight loss decreases white adipose tissue, hepatic steatosis, improves insulin sensitivity, and also decreases inflammatory markers.[122]

Pharmacologic Interventions

Antiobesity

Currently there is only one medication that has been approved for weight reduction. Orlistat is a lipase inhibitor that blocks the absorption of long-chain fatty acids and cholesterol from small intestine. Harrison et al evaluated the antiobesity effect of orlistat in a group of adults with biopsy-proven NASH.[123] They demonstrated that orlistat treatment decreased BMI and significantly improved biochemical parameters associated with NASH. Other medications including sibutramine (a serotonin and norepinephrine reuptake inhibitor)[124] and rimonabant (cannabinoid receptor type 1 antagonist) have been shown to result in weight reduction and improvement in biochemical markers and sonographic evidence of hepatic steatosis.[125] However, the latter medications are no longer approved for management of obesity due to undesirable side-effects and safety concerns. Nevertheless, randomized clinical trials are needed to determine the safety and efficacy of antiobesity medications in patients with NAFLD.

Attenuation of Insulin Resistance

It has been documented that insulin resistance plays a significant role in the pathophysiology of NASH. Indeed, clinical features of metabolic syndrome and insulin resistance are present in approximately 66% of patients with NAFLD.[52] Pharmacologic intervention is aimed at attenuating insulin resistance. Metformin and thiazolinediones have been evaluated for treatment of insulin resistance in individuals with NAFLD or NASH.

Metformin

Metformin is a biguanide that decreases hyperinsulinemia and enhances insulin sensitivity by reducing hepatic glucose output and increasing the peripheral glucose uptake by skeletal muscle and fatty acid oxidation. Indeed, metformin is a well-established oral hypoglycemic agent in the treatment of adults and adolescents with type 2 diabetes mellitus and other conditions associated with insulin resistance.[126] In pediatric obese patients with insulin resistance, metformin has also been shown to promote weight loss.[127, 128] It was observed that short-term use of metformin is well tolerated by obese children and that it has a beneficial effect on BMI. In nondiabetic adults, small trials use of high-dose metformin (2 gm daily) along with weight reducing diet or vitamin E 800 IU observed that metformin treatment resulted in reduction in serum ALT with improved steatosis, inflammation and fibrosis compared to vitamin E.[129] However, another study showed that high-dose metformin improved biochemical parameters after 3 months without significant difference at one year.[130] In a group of obese adolescents, metformin therapy (1 gm daily) resulted only in reduced BMI and visceral adiposity compared to placebo group without significant difference in serum transaminases and sonographic evidence of steatosis between the two groups after one year.[131] Recently, Lavine et al reported the results of a large multicenter trial [The Treatment of NAFLD in Children (TONIC) trial] assessing the efficacy of metformin and vitamin E. They reported that neither vitamin E nor metformin (1 gm daily) was superior to placebo in reducing sustained reduction in serum transaminases in pediatric NAFLD patients.[132] Indeed, metformin treatment only improved hepatocellular ballooning without significant histological improvements compared to placebo over 96 weeks. On the other hand, vitamin E treatment resulted in histological improvements in those with NASH or borderline NASH. It is possible that the lack of significant treatment effect on liver transaminases and liver steatosis in these pediatric studies may have been due to the lower dose of metformin used. In addition, poor adherence to metformin dosing among this pediatric cohort may have been due to dose-dependent nausea, vomiting and diarrhea in some patients cannot be ruled out. In addition, Fu et al observed that metformin may have anti-inflammatory and lipolytic effects mediated through adipocytokines.[133] Therefore, further clinical trials involving larger randomized placebo-controlled cohorts for the evaluation of low and high-dose metformin treatment effect on metabolic and inflammation biomarkers as well as steatosis are needed.

Thiazolidinediones

Thiazolidinediones are oral antidiabetic medications that have been evaluated for treatment of NASH. They bind to peroxisome proliferator-activated receptor gamma (PPAR-γ) and enhance insulin sensitivity by various mechanisms. They have been shown to stimulate free fatty acid oxidation and increase plasma adiponectin and leptin concentrations.[134, 135] Several studies have assessed the efficacy of thiazolidinediones in adult patients with NASH. It has been shown that use of rosiglitazone in biopsy-proven NASH improved insulin resistance, transaminases, and liver histology after 48 weeks of treatment.[136] However, the improvement in liver transaminases reversed in association with weight gain. Ratziu et al demonstrated that the use of rosiglitazone in patients with NASH improved steatosis and insulin sensitivity and reduced transaminase but it resulted in significant weight gain.[137] To date, the efficacy and safety of thiazolinediones have not been evaluated in pediatric NAFLD or NASH. Since this class of drug has been shown to increase the cardiovascular risks in adults, caution is advised in the long term use of thiazolinediones in patients with NASH.[138]

Antioxidants

Oxidative stress plays a major role in the multi-hit hypothesis of NAFLD. Antioxidants such as vitamin E, vitamin C, and ursodeoxycholic acid (UDCA) are potentially hepatoprotective agents that have been evaluated in clinical studies. These compounds may slow the progression of steatosis to steatohepatitis by reducing oxidative damage to hepatocytes. Two treatment trials have tested the efficacy of supplemental vitamin E, or vitamin E and C in normalizing serum ALT and AST levels.[139, 140] Recently, the TONIC trial observed that vitamin E treatment resulted in histological improvements in those with NASH or borderline NASH.[132]

Currently, the hepatoprotective effects of ursodeoxycholic acid (UDCA) with or without vitamin E are being evaluated for medical management of NAFLD by several investigators. In a small pilot study of adults with NASH, Laurin et al demonstrated that UDCA treatment at daily doses of 13 to 15 mg reduced steatosis and serum liver transaminases after 2 years.[141] However, the hepatoprotective effect of UDCA was evaluated by a randomized, double-blind, placebo-controlled in a large cohort of adult patients with NASH while medical treatment was apparently well tolerated, no biochemical or histological improvements were observed.[142]

Bariatric Surgery

Bariatric surgery has been proposed as a potential intervention since obesity is accompanied by NASH.[143] Adolescents are increasingly undergoing surgical treatment of obesity, though the guidelines for eligibility are not standardized.[144-146] Recently, the use of laproscopic adjustable gastric banding compared with lifestyle intervention was reported to result in a greater percentage achieving a loss of 50% of excess weight in a group of severely obese adolescents.[147] This interventional approach may be preferable to other surgical procedures in the management of adolescents with NASH. It is yet to be determined whether NASH should be considered a major or minor criterion for bariatric surgery. Alternatively, the presence of underlying cirrhosis may disqualify a patient being a surgical candidate, or conversely, facilitate the decision to proceed with surgery. Children with a clinical diagnosis of NAFLD are often younger and less obese than adolescents undergoing surgical treatment of obesity.[15, 51, 77] Therefore, bariatric surgery screening criteria for individuals with NAFLD may need to be altered in the context of the severity of steatohepatitis. While bariatric surgery in adults with NAFLD has shown to improve histology,[148, 149] similar outcome data in adolescents are needed to establish guidelines for the use of bariatric surgery in this cohort.

Liver Transplantation for NASH

Children and adolescents with NAFLD may develop end-stage liver disease with the consequent need for liver transplantation. NAFLD in children seen in a tertiary care center may be associated with a significantly shorter survival as compared to the general population Feldtein et al followed a group of 66 pediatric patients for period of 20 years.[65] Two patients who were followed for an average of 11 years underwent liver transplantation due to cirrhosis with end-stage liver disease and hepatopulmonary syndrome as young adults.

In adults, fatty liver is common after liver transplantation for cryptogenic cirrhosis or NASH but is twice as common in the latter group. Yalamanchili et al suggested that some cryptogenic cirrhosis, but perhaps not all, is caused by NASH.[150] Post-transplant NASH is unusual, and steatosis appears to be a prerequisite. Similarly, hepatic steatosis and even recurrent NASH has been reported in post-transplant younger patients.[65] Nevertheless, advanced fibrosis is uncommon, and survival is the same as that of patients who undergo transplantation for other causes.[150]

Conclusion

NAFLD is the most common cause of chronic liver disease in children, with some few cases progressing to NASH. In some children, NASH progresses to advanced fibrosis and even cirrhosis. The epidemic of obesity and its metabolic consequences have played a significant role in the development of NAFLD and NASH. The growing number of cases of NASH represents a largely unknown public health crisis. Its prevalence and the overall liver-related mortality are expected to increase with rising rates of obesity and type 2 diabetes in adolescents. The exact genetic and environmental factors influencing the development of NASH remain elusive. It is important to diagnose NAFLD and identify patients with NASH [151]. There are currently no definitive non-invasive tests for diagnosis of NASH. Therefore, liver biopsy remains the only reliable tool for the diagnosis and staging of NASH. It is critical to determine the natural history of pediatric NAFLD and NASH and their corresponding histological features. Current interventions for NAFLD include weight loss through lifestyle changes and treatment for insulin resistance and the other components of metabolic syndrome. However, the effectiveness of these treatment modalities needs to be further evaluated through rigorous double-blind, controlled trials. Future treatment trials should focus on treatment of children and adolescents with steatohepatitis. It is critical to educate pediatric physicians regarding the prevalence of NAFLD and NASH among children and adolescents in order to prevent morbidity associated with NASH and progression to cirrhosis and end-stage liver disease.

References

[1] Adler M, Schaffner F. *Fatty liver hepatitis and cirrhosis in obese patients.* The American journal of medicine. 1979 Nov;67(5):811-6.

[2] Ludwig J, Viggiano TR, McGill DB, Oh BJ. *Nonalcoholic steatohepatitis: Mayo Clinic experiences with a hitherto unnamed disease.* Mayo Clinic proceedings. 1980 Jul;55(7):434-8.

[3] Patton HM, Sirlin C, Behling C, Middleton M, Schwimmer JB, Lavine JE. *Pediatric nonalcoholic fatty liver disease: a critical appraisal of current data and implications for future research.* Journal of pediatric gastroenterology and nutrition. 2006 Oct;43(4):413-27.

[4] Abrams S. Fatty Liver Disease. In: Colin D. Rudolph M, PhD, ed. *Rudolph's Pediatrics.* 22 edition ed. New York: McGraw-Hill 2011:1524-5.

[5] McCullough AJ. *Pathophysiology of nonalcoholic steatohepatitis. Journal of clinical gastroenterology.* 2006 Mar;40 Suppl 1:S17-29.

[6] Iacobellis A, Marcellini M, Andriulli A, Perri F, Leandro G, Devito R, et al. *Non invasive evaluation of liver fibrosis in paediatric patients with nonalcoholic steatohepatitis.* World J Gastroenterol. 2006 Dec 28;12(48):7821-5.

[7] Schwimmer JB, Deutsch R, Kahen T, Lavine JE, Stanley C, Behling C. *Prevalence of fatty liver in children and adolescents.* Pediatrics. 2006 Oct;118(4):1388-93.

[8] Tominaga K, Kurata JH, Chen YK, Fujimoto E, Miyagawa S, Abe I, et al. *Prevalence of fatty liver in Japanese children and relationship to obesity. An epidemiological ultrasonographic survey.* Digestive diseases and sciences. 1995 Sep;40(9):2002-9.

[9] Franzese A, Vajro P, Argenziano A, Puzziello A, Iannucci MP, Saviano MC, et al. *Liver involvement in obese children. Ultrasonography and liver enzyme levels at diagnosis and during follow-up in an Italian population.* Digestive diseases and sciences. 1997 Jul;42(7):1428-32.

[10] Chan DF, Li AM, Chu WC, Chan MH, Wong EM, Liu EK, et al. *Hepatic steatosis in obese Chinese children.* Int J Obes Relat Metab Disord. 2004 Oct;28(10):1257-63.

[11] Denzer C, Thiere D, Muche R, Koenig W, Mayer H, Kratzer W, et al. *Gender-specific prevalences of fatty liver in obese children and adolescents: roles of body fat distribution, sex steroids, and insulin*

resistance. The Journal of clinical endocrinology and metabolism. 2009 Oct;94(10):3872-81.

[12] Adams LA, Sanderson S, Lindor KD, Angulo P. *The histological course of nonalcoholic fatty liver disease: a longitudinal study of 103 patients with sequential liver biopsies.* Journal of hepatology. 2005 Jan;42(1):132-8.

[13] Brunt EM, Neuschwander-Tetri BA, Oliver D, Wehmeier KR, Bacon BR. *Nonalcoholic steatohepatitis: histologic features and clinical correlations with 30 blinded biopsy specimens.* Human pathology. 2004 Sep;35(9):1070-82.

[14] Larter CZ, Chitturi S, Heydet D, Farrell GC. *A fresh look at NASH pathogenesis. Part 1: the metabolic movers*. Journal of gastroenterology and hepatology. Apr;25(4):672-90.

[15] Schwimmer JB, Behling C, Newbury R, Deutsch R, Nievergelt C, Schork NJ, et al. *Histopathology of pediatric nonalcoholic fatty liver disease.* Hepatology (Baltimore, Md. 2005 Sep;42(3):641-9.

[16] Ogden CL, Carroll MD, Curtin LR, Lamb MM, Flegal KM. *Prevalence of high body mass index in US children and adolescents, 2007-2008.* Jama. Jan 20;303(3):242-9.

[17] Sanyal AJ, Campbell-Sargent C, Mirshahi F, Rizzo WB, Contos MJ, Sterling RK, et al. *Nonalcoholic steatohepatitis: association of insulin resistance and mitochondrial abnormalitie*s. Gastroenterology. 2001 Apr;120(5):1183-92.

[18] Marchesini G, Brizi M, Bianchi G, Tomassetti S, Bugianesi E, Lenzi M, et al. *Nonalcoholic fatty liver disease: a feature of the metabolic syndrome.* Diabetes. 2001 Aug;50(8):1844-50.

[19] Dixon JB, Bhathal PS, O'Brien PE. *Nonalcoholic fatty liver disease: predictors of nonalcoholic steatohepatitis and liver fibrosis in the severely obese.* Gastroenterology. 2001 Jul;121(1):91-100.

[20] Ratziu V, Giral P, Charlotte F, Bruckert E, Thibault V, Theodorou I, et al. *Liver fibrosis in overweight patients.* Gastroenterology. 2000 Jun;118(6):1117-23.

[21] Day CP, James OF. *Steatohepatitis: a tale of two "hits"?* Gastroenterology. 1998 Apr;114(4):842-5.

[22] Vega GL, Chandalia M, Szczepaniak LS, Grundy SM. *Metabolic correlates of nonalcoholic fatty liver in women and men.* Hepatology (Baltimore, Md. 2007 Sep;46(3):716-22.

[23] Fan JG, Farrell GC. *VAT fat is bad for the liver, SAT fat is not!* Journal of gastroenterology and hepatology. 2008 Jun;23(6):829-32.

[24] Friedman J. *Fat in all the wrong places.* Nature. 2002 Jan 17;415(6869):268-9.

[25] Park EJ, Lee JH, Yu GY, He G, Ali SR, Holzer RG, et al. *Dietary and genetic obesity promote liver inflammation and tumorigenesis by enhancing IL-6 and TNF expression.* Cell. Jan 22;140(2):197-208.

[26] Makino T, Noguchi Y, Yoshikawa T, Doi C, Nomura K. *Circulating interleukin 6 concentrations and insulin resistance in patients with cancer.* The British journal of surgery. 1998 Dec;85(12):1658-62.

[27] Fernandez-Real JM, Vayreda M, Richart C, Gutierrez C, Broch M, Vendrell J, et al. *Circulating interleukin 6 levels, blood pressure, and insulin sensitivity in apparently healthy men and women. The Journal of clinical endocrinology and metabolism.* 2001 Mar;86(3):1154-9.

[28] Kern PA, Saghizadeh M, Ong JM, Bosch RJ, Deem R, Simsolo RB. *The expression of tumor necrosis factor in human adipose tissue. Regulation by obesity, weight loss, and relationship to lipoprotein lipase.* The Journal of clinical investigation. 1995 May;95(5):2111-9.

[29] Diehl AM, Goodman Z, Ishak KG. *Alcohollike liver disease in nonalcoholics. A clinical and histologic comparison with alcohol-induced liver injury.* Gastroenterology. 1988 Oct;95(4):1056-62.

[30] Burgert TS, Taksali SE, Dziura J, Goodman TR, Yeckel CW, *Papademetris X, et al. Alanine aminotransferase levels and fatty liver in childhood obesity: associations with insulin resistance, adiponectin, and visceral fat.* The Journal of clinical endocrinology and metabolism. 2006 Nov;91(11):4287-94.

[31] Nadeau KJ, Klingensmith G, Zeitler P. *Type 2 diabetes in children is frequently associated with elevated alanine aminotransferase.* Journal of pediatric gastroenterology and nutrition. 2005 Jul;41(1):94-8.

[32] Fraser A, Longnecker MP, Lawlor DA. *Prevalence of elevated alanine aminotransferase among US adolescents and associated factors: NHANES 1999-2004.* Gastroenterology. 2007 Dec;133(6):1814-20.

[33] Takahashi Y, Fukusato T. *Pediatric nonalcoholic fatty liver disease: overview with emphasis on histology.* World J Gastroenterol. Nov 14;16(42):5280-5.

[34] Sundaram SS, Zeitler P, Nadeau K. *The metabolic syndrome and nonalcoholic fatty liver disease in children.* Current opinion in pediatrics. 2009 Aug;21(4):529-35.

[35] Lopez-Alvarenga JC, Montesinos-Cabrera RA, Velazquez-Alva C, Gonzalez-Barranco J. *Short stature is related to high body fat*

composition despite body mass index in a Mexican population. Archives of medical research. 2003 Mar-Apr;34(2):137-40.

[36] Marra F. *NASH: are genes blowing the hits?* Journal of hepatology. 2004 May;40(5):853-6.

[37] Namikawa C, Shu-Ping Z, Vyselaar JR, Nozaki Y, Nemoto Y, Ono M, et al. *Polymorphisms of microsomal triglyceride transfer protein gene and manganese superoxide dismutase gene in non-alcoholic steatohepatitis.* Journal of hepatology. 2004 May;40(5):781-6.

[38] Tokushige K, Yatsuji S, Hashimoto E, Kabutake A, Tobari M, Taniai M, et al. *Familial aggregation in patients with non-alcoholic steatohepatitis.* Internal medicine (Tokyo, Japan). 2008;47(5):405-10.

[39] Song J, da Costa KA, Fischer LM, Kohlmeier M, Kwock L, Wang S, et al. *Polymorphism of the PEMT gene and susceptibility to nonalcoholic fatty liver disease (NAFLD).* Faseb J. 2005 Aug;19(10):1266-71.

[40] Dong H, Wang J, Li C, Hirose A, Nozaki Y, Takahashi M, et al. *The phosphatidylethanolamine N-methyltransferase gene V175M single nucleotide polymorphism confers the susceptibility to NASH in Japanese population.* Journal of hepatology. 2007 May;46(5):915-20.

[41] Tokushige K, Takakura M, Tsuchiya-Matsushita N, Taniai M, Hashimoto E, Shiratori K. *Influence of TNF gene polymorphisms in Japanese patients with NASH and simple steatosis.* Journal of hepatology. 2007 Jun;46(6):1104-10.

[42] Schwimmer JB, Deutsch R, Rauch JB, Behling C, Newbury R, Lavine JE. *Obesity, insulin resistance, and other clinicopathological correlates of pediatric nonalcoholic fatty liver disease.* The Journal of pediatrics. 2003 Oct;143(4):500-5.

[43] Tarantino G, Saldalamacchia G, Conca P, Arena A. *Non-alcoholic fatty liver disease: further expression of the metabolic syndrome.* Journal of gastroenterology and hepatology. 2007 Mar;22(3):293-303.

[44] Fierbinteanu-Braticevici C, Baicus C, Tribus L, Papacocea R. *Predictive factors for nonalcoholic steatohepatitis (NASH) in patients with nonalcoholic fatty liver disease (NAFLD).* J Gastrointestin Liver Dis. Jun;20(2):153-9.

[45] Assy N, Schlesinger S, Hussein O. *Elevated plasma protein C levels correlate with the presence of fatty liver (NASH and NAFLD).* Gut. 2005 May;54(5):729.

[46] Yoneda M, Mawatari H, Fujita K, Iida H, Yonemitsu K, Kato S, et al. *High-sensitivity C-reactive protein is an independent clinical feature of*

nonalcoholic steatohepatitis (NASH) and also of the severity of fibrosis in NASH. Journal of gastroenterology. 2007 Jul;42(7):573-82.

[47] Powell EE, Cooksley WG, Hanson R, Searle J, Halliday JW, Powell LW. *The natural history of nonalcoholic steatohepatitis: a follow-up study of forty-two patients for up to 21 years.* Hepatology (Baltimore, Md. 1990 Jan;11(1):74-80.

[48] Loguercio C, De Girolamo V, de Sio I, Tuccillo C, Ascione A, Baldi F, et al. *Non-alcoholic fatty liver disease in an area of southern Italy: main clinical, histological, and pathophysiological aspects.* Journal of hepatology. 2001 Nov;35(5):568-74.

[49] Teli MR, James OF, Burt AD, Bennett MK, Day CP. *The natural history of nonalcoholic fatty liver: a follow-up study.* Hepatology (Baltimore, Md. 1995 Dec;22(6):1714-9.

[50] Liou I, Kowdley KV. *Natural history of nonalcoholic steatohepatitis.* Journal of clinical gastroenterology. 2006 Mar;40 Suppl 1:S11-6.

[51] Nobili V, Marcellini M, Devito R, Ciampalini P, Piemonte F, Comparcola D, et al. *NAFLD in children: a prospective clinical-pathological study and effect of lifestyle advice.* Hepatology (Baltimore, Md. 2006 Aug;44(2):458-65.

[52] Manco M, Marcellini M, Devito R, Comparcola D, Sartorelli MR, Nobili V. *Metabolic syndrome and liver histology in paediatric non-alcoholic steatohepatitis.* International journal of obesity (2005). 2008 Feb;32(2):381-7.

[53] Marchesini G, Bugianesi E, Forlani G, Cerrelli F, Lenzi M, Manini R, et al. N*onalcoholic fatty liver, steatohepatitis, and the metabolic syndrome.* Hepatology (Baltimore, Md. 2003 Apr;37(4):917-23.

[54] Contos MJ, Cales W, Sterling RK, Luketic VA, Shiffman ML, Mills AS, et al. *Development of nonalcoholic fatty liver disease after orthotopic liver transplantation for cryptogenic cirrhosis.* Liver Transpl. 2001 Apr;7(4):363-73.

[55] Drenick EJ, Fisler J, Johnson D. *Hepatic steatosis after intestinal bypass--prevention and reversal by metronidazole, irrespective of protein-calorie malnutrition.* Gastroenterology. 1982 Mar;82(3):535-48.

[56] Luyckx FH, Desaive C, Thiry A, Dewe W, Scheen AJ, Gielen JE, et al. *Liver abnormalities in severely obese subjects: effect of drastic weight loss after gastroplasty.* Int J Obes Relat Metab Disord. 1998 Mar;22(3):222-6.

[57] Kinugasa A, Tsunamoto K, Furukawa N, Sawada T, Kusunoki T, Shimada N. *Fatty liver and its fibrous changes found in simple obesity of*

children. Journal of pediatric gastroenterology and nutrition. 1984 Jun;3(3):408-14.

[58] Molleston JP, White F, Teckman J, Fitzgerald JF. *Obese children with steatohepatitis can develop cirrhosis in childhood.* The American journal of gastroenterology. 2002 Sep;97(9):2460-2.

[59] Suzuki D, Hashimoto E, Kaneda K, Tokushige K, Shiratori K. *Liver failure caused by non-alcoholic steatohepatitis in an obese young male.* Journal of gastroenterology and hepatology. 2005 Feb;20(2):327-9.

[60] Harrison SA, Torgerson S, Hayashi PH. *The natural history of nonalcoholic fatty liver disease: a clinical histopathological study.* The American journal of gastroenterology. 2003 Sep;98(9):2042-7.

[61] Fassio E, Alvarez E, Dominguez N, Landeira G, Longo C. *Natural history of nonalcoholic steatohepatitis: a longitudinal study of repeat liver biopsies.* Hepatology (Baltimore, Md. 2004 Oct;40(4):820-6.

[62] Ekstedt M, Franzen LE, Mathiesen UL, Thorelius L, Holmqvist M, Bodemar G, et al. *Long-term follow-up of patients with NAFLD and elevated liver enzymes.* Hepatology (Baltimore, Md. 2006 Oct;44(4):865-73.

[63] Angulo P. *GI epidemiology: nonalcoholic fatty liver disease.* Alimentary pharmacology and therapeutics. 2007 Apr 15;25(8):883-9.

[64] Clark JM. *The epidemiology of nonalcoholic fatty liver disease in adults.* Journal of clinical gastroenterology. 2006 Mar;40 Suppl 1:S5-10.

[65] Feldstein AE, Charatcharoenwitthaya P, Treeprasertsuk S, Benson JT, Enders FB, Angulo P. *The natural history of non-alcoholic fatty liver disease in children: a follow-up study for up to 20 years.* Gut. 2009 Nov;58(11):1538-44.

[66] Garcia-Monzon C, Martin-Perez E, Iacono OL, Fernandez-Bermejo M, Majano PL, Apolinario A, et al. *Characterization of pathogenic and prognostic factors of nonalcoholic steatohepatitis associated with obesity.* Journal of hepatology. 2000 Nov;33(5):716-24.

[67] Matteoni CA, Younossi ZM, Gramlich T, Boparai N, Liu YC, McCullough AJ. *Nonalcoholic fatty liver disease: a spectrum of clinical and pathological severity.* Gastroenterology. 1999 Jun;116(6):1413-9.

[68] Lee RG. *Nonalcoholic steatohepatitis: a study of 49 patients.* Human pathology. 1989 Jun;20(6):594-8.

[69] Evans CD, Oien KA, MacSween RN, Mills PR. *Non-alcoholic steatohepatitis: a common cause of progressive chronic liver injury?* Journal of clinical pathology. 2002 Sep;55(9):689-92.

[70] Dam-Larsen S, Franzmann M, Andersen IB, Christoffersen P, Jensen LB, Sorensen TI, et al. *Long term prognosis of fatty liver: risk of chronic liver disease and death.* Gut. 2004 May;53(5):750-5.

[71] Rafiq N, Bai C, Fang Y, Srishord M, McCullough A, Gramlich T, et al. *Long-term follow-up of patients with nonalcoholic fatty liver.* Clin Gastroenterol Hepatol. 2009 Feb;7(2):234-8.

[72] Baldridge AD, Perez-Atayde AR, Graeme-Cook F, Higgins L, Lavine JE. *Idiopathic steatohepatitis in childhood: a multicenter retrospective study.* The Journal of pediatrics. 1995 Nov;127(5):700-4.

[73] Jonas MM, Krawczuk LE, Kim HB, Lillehei C, Perez-Atayde A. *Rapid recurrence of nonalcoholic fatty liver disease after transplantation in a child with hypopituitarism and hepatopulmonary syndrome.* Liver Transpl. 2005 Jan;11(1):108-10.

[74] Jankowska I, Socha P, Pawlowska J, Teisseyre M, Gliwicz D, Czubkowski P, et al. *Recurrence of non-alcoholic steatohepatitis after liver transplantation in a 13-yr-old boy.* Pediatric transplantation. 2007 Nov;11(7):796-8.

[75] Adams LA, Feldstein A, Lindor KD, Angulo P. *Nonalcoholic fatty liver disease among patients with hypothalamic and pituitary dysfunction.* Hepatology (Baltimore, Md. 2004 Apr;39(4):909-14.

[76] Rashid M, Roberts EA. *Nonalcoholic steatohepatitis in children.* Journal of pediatric gastroenterology and nutrition. 2000 Jan;30(1):48-53.

[77] Patton HM, Lavine JE, Van Natta ML, Schwimmer JB, Kleiner D, Molleston J. *Clinical correlates of histopathology in pediatric nonalcoholic steatohepatitis.* Gastroenterology. 2008 Dec;135(6):1961-71 e2.

[78] Schwimmer JB, McGreal N, Deutsch R, Finegold MJ, Lavine JE. *Influence of gender, race, and ethnicity on suspected fatty liver in obese adolescents.* Pediatrics. 2005 May;115(5):e561-5.

[79] Manton ND, Lipsett J, Moore DJ, Davidson GP, Bourne AJ, Couper RT. *Non-alcoholic steatohepatitis in children and adolescents.* The Medical journal of Australia. 2000 Nov 6;173(9):476-9.

[80] Cook JS, Hoffman RP, Stene MA, Hansen JR. *Effects of maturational stage on insulin sensitivity during puberty.* The Journal of clinical endocrinology and metabolism. 1993 Sep;77(3):725-30.

[81] Roemmich JN, Clark PA, Lusk M, Friel A, Weltman A, Epstein LH, et al. *Pubertal alterations in growth and body composition. VI. Pubertal insulin resistance: relation to adiposity, body fat distribution and hormone release.* Int J Obes Relat Metab Disord. 2002 May;26(5):701-9.

[82] Goran MI, Gower BA. *Longitudinal study on pubertal insulin resistance.* Diabetes. 2001 Nov;50(11):2444-50.

[83] Williamson RM, Price JF, Glancy S, Perry E, Nee LD, Hayes PC, et al. *Prevalence of and risk factors for hepatic steatosis and nonalcoholic Fatty liver disease in people with type 2 diabetes: the edinburgh type 2 diabetes study.* Diabetes care. May;34(5):1139-44.

[84] Stranges S, Dorn JM, Muti P, Freudenheim JL, Farinaro E, Russell M, et al. *Body fat distribution, relative weight, and liver enzyme levels: a population-based study.* Hepatology (Baltimore, Md. 2004 Mar;39(3):754-63.

[85] Ellis KJ. *Body composition of a young, multiethnic, male population. The American journal of clinical nutrition. 1997 Dec;66(6):1323-31.*

[86] Patton HM, Yates K, Unalp-Arida A, Behling CA, Huang TT, Rosenthal P, et al. *Association between metabolic syndrome and liver histology among children with nonalcoholic Fatty liver disease.* The American journal of gastroenterology. Sep;105(9):2093-102.

[87] Roberts EA. *Pediatric nonalcoholic fatty liver disease (NAFLD): a "growing" problem?* Journal of hepatology. 2007 Jun;46(6):1133-42.

[88] Bacon BR, Farahvash MJ, Janney CG, Neuschwander-Tetri BA. *Nonalcoholic steatohepatitis: an expanded clinical entity.* Gastroenterology. 1994 Oct;107(4):1103-9.

[89] Nobili V, Parkes J, Bottazzo G, Marcellini M, Cross R, Newman D, et al. *Performance of ELF serum markers in predicting fibrosis stage in pediatric non-alcoholic fatty liver disease.* Gastroenterology. 2009 Jan;136(1):160-7.

[90] Lavine JE, Schwimmer JB. *Nonalcoholic fatty liver disease in the pediatric population.* Clinics in liver disease. 2004 Aug;8(3):549-58, viii-ix.

[91] Barlow SE. *Expert committee recommendations regarding the prevention, assessment, and treatment of child and adolescent overweight and obesity: summary report.* Pediatrics. 2007 Dec;120 Suppl 4:S164-92.

[92] Kang YH, Min HK, Son SM, Kim IJ, Kim YK. *The association of serum gamma glutamyltransferase with components of the metabolic syndrome in the Korean adults.* Diabetes research and clinical practice. 2007 Aug;77(2):306-13.

[93] Lee DH, Ha MH, Kim JH, Christiani DC, Gross MD, Steffes M, et al. *Gamma-glutamyltransferase and diabetes--a 4 year follow-up study.* Diabetologia. 2003 Mar;46(3):359-64.

[94] Kim DJ, Noh JH, Cho NH, Lee BW, Choi YH, Jung JH, et al. *Serum gamma-glutamyltransferase within its normal concentration range is related to the presence of diabetes and cardiovascular risk factors.* Diabet Med. 2005 Sep;22(9):1134-40.

[95] Cotler SJ, Kanji K, Keshavarzian A, Jensen DM, Jakate S. *Prevalence and significance of autoantibodies in patients with non-alcoholic steatohepatitis.* Journal of clinical gastroenterology. 2004 Oct;38(9):801-4.

[96] Mehta SR, Thomas EL, Bell JD, Johnston DG, Taylor-Robinson SD. *Non-invasive means of measuring hepatic fat conten*t. World J Gastroenterol. 2008 Jun 14;14(22):3476-83.

[97] Siegelman ES, Rosen MA. *Imaging of hepatic steatosis.* Seminars in liver disease. 2001;21(1):71-80.

[98] *Strauss S, Gavish E, Gottlieb P, Katsnelson L. Interobserver and intraobserver variability in the sonographic assessment of fatty liver.* Ajr. 2007 Dec;189(6):W320-3.

[99] Joseph AE, Saverymuttu SH, al-Sam S, Cook MG, Maxwell JD. *Comparison of liver histology with ultrasonography in assessing diffuse parenchymal liver disease.* Clinical radiology. 1991 Jan;43(1):26-31.

[100] Fishbein M, Castro F, Cheruku S, Jain S, Webb B, Gleason T, et al. *Hepatic MRI for fat quantitation: its relationship to fat morphology, diagnosis, and ultrasound.* Journal of clinical gastroenterology. 2005 Aug;39(7):619-25.

[101] Ricci C, Longo R, Gioulis E, Bosco M, Pollesello P, Masutti F, et al. *Noninvasive in vivo quantitative assessment of fat content in human liver.* Journal of hepatology. 1997 Jul;27(1):108-13.

[102] Park SH, Kim PN, Kim KW, Lee SW, Yoon SE, Park SW, et al. *Macrovesicular hepatic steatosis in living liver donors: use of CT for quantitative and qualitative assessment.* Radiology. 2006 Apr;239(1):105-12.

[103] Fishbein MH, Miner M, Mogren C, Chalekson J. *The spectrum of fatty liver in obese children and the relationship of serum aminotransferases to severity of steatosis.* Journal of pediatric gastroenterology and nutrition. 2003 Jan;36(1):54-61.

[104] Pacifico L, Celestre M, Anania C, Paolantonio P, Chiesa C, Laghi A. *MRI and ultrasound for hepatic fat quantification:relationships to clinical and metabolic characteristics of pediatric nonalcoholic fatty liver disease.* Acta Paediatr. 2007 Apr;96(4):542-7.

[105] Szczepaniak LS, Nurenberg P, Leonard D, Browning JD, Reingold JS, Grundy S, et al. *Magnetic resonance spectroscopy to measure hepatic triglyceride content: prevalence of hepatic steatosis in the general population*. American journal of physiology. 2005 Feb;288(2):E462-8.

[106] Foucher J, Chanteloup E, Vergniol J, Castera L, Le Bail B, Adhoute X, et al. *Diagnosis of cirrhosis by transient elastography (FibroScan): a prospective study*. Gut. 2006 Mar;55(3):403-8.

[107] Ziol M, Handra-Luca A, Kettaneh A, Christidis C, Mal F, Kazemi F, et al. *Noninvasive assessment of liver fibrosis by measurement of stiffness in patients with chronic hepatitis C*. Hepatology (Baltimore, Md. 2005 Jan;41(1):48-54.

[108] Younossi ZM, Gramlich T, Liu YC, Matteoni C, Petrelli M, Goldblum J, et al. *Nonalcoholic fatty liver disease: assessment of variability in pathologic interpretations*. Mod Pathol. 1998 Jun;11(6):560-5.

[109] Kleiner DE, Brunt EM, Van Natta M, Behling C, Contos MJ, Cummings OW, et al. *Design and validation of a histological scoring system for nonalcoholic fatty liver disease*. Hepatology (Baltimore, Md. 2005 Jun;41(6):1313-21.

[110] Baranova A, Younossi ZM. *The future is around the corner: Noninvasive diagnosis of progressive nonalcoholic steatohepatitis*. Hepatology (Baltimore, Md. 2008 Feb;47(2):373-5.

[111] Ong JP, Younossi ZM. *Approach to the diagnosis and treatment of nonalcoholic fatty liver disease*. Clinics in liver disease. 2005 Nov;9(4):617-34, vi.

[112] Wieckowska A, McCullough AJ, Feldstein AE. *Noninvasive diagnosis and monitoring of nonalcoholic steatohepatitis: present and future*. Hepatology (Baltimore, Md. 2007 Aug;46(2):582-9.

[113] Wieckowska A, Zein NN, Yerian LM, Lopez AR, McCullough AJ, Feldstein AE. *In vivo assessment of liver cell apoptosis as a novel biomarker of disease severity in nonalcoholic fatty liver disease*. Hepatology (Baltimore, Md. 2006 Jul;44(1):27-33.

[114] Younossi ZM, Jarrar M, Nugent C, Randhawa M, Afendy M, Stepanova M, et al. *A novel diagnostic biomarker panel for obesity-related nonalcoholic steatohepatitis (NASH)*. Obesity surgery. 2008 Nov;18(11):1430-7.

[115] Bedogni G, Bellentani S, Miglioli L, Masutti F, Passalacqua M, Castiglione A, et al. *The Fatty Liver Index: a simple and accurate predictor of hepatic steatosis in the general population*. BMC gastroenterology. 2006;6:33.

[116] Ratziu V, Massard J, Charlotte F, Messous D, Imbert-Bismut F, Bonyhay L, et al. *Diagnostic value of biochemical markers (FibroTest-FibroSURE) for the prediction of liver fibrosis in patients with non-alcoholic fatty liver disease*. BMC gastroenterology. 2006;6:6.

[117] Poynard T, Ratziu V, Naveau S, Thabut D, Charlotte F, Messous D, et al. *The diagnostic value of biomarkers (SteatoTest) for the prediction of liver steatosis.* Comparative hepatology. 2005;4:10.

[118] Nobili V, Manco M, Devito R, Di Ciommo V, Comparcola D, Sartorelli MR, et al. *Lifestyle intervention and antioxidant therapy in children with nonalcoholic fatty liver disease: a randomized, controlled trial.* Hepatology (Baltimore, Md. 2008 Jul;48(1):119-28.

[119] Stewart KJ, Bacher AC, Turner K, Lim JG, Hees PS, Shapiro EP, et al. *Exercise and risk factors associated with metabolic syndrome in older adults.* American journal of preventive medicine. 2005 Jan;28(1):9-18.

[120] Palmer M, Schaffner F. *Effect of weight reduction on hepatic abnormalities in overweight patients.* Gastroenterology. 1990 Nov;99(5):1408-13.

[121] Ueno T, Sugawara H, Sujaku K, Hashimoto O, Tsuji R, Tamaki S, et al. *Therapeutic effects of restricted diet and exercise in obese patients with fatty liver.* Journal of hepatology. 1997 Jul;27(1):103-7.

[122] Rafiq N, Younossi ZM. *Effects of weight loss on nonalcoholic fatty liver disease.* Seminars in liver disease. 2008 Nov;28(4):427-33.

[123] Harrison SA, Fincke C, Helinski D, Torgerson S, Hayashi P. *A pilot study of orlistat treatment in obese, non-alcoholic steatohepatitis patients.* Alimentary pharmacology and therapeutics. 2004 Sep 15;20(6):623-8.

[124] Sabuncu T, Nazligul Y, Karaoglanoglu M, Ucar E, Kilic FB. *The effects of sibutramine and orlistat on the ultrasonographic findings, insulin resistance and liver enzyme levels in obese patients with non-alcoholic steatohepatitis.* Romanian journal of gastroenterology. 2003 Sep;12(3):189-92.

[125] Gary-Bobo M, Elachouri G, Gallas JF, Janiak P, Marini P, Ravinet-Trillou C, et al. *Rimonabant reduces obesity-associated hepatic steatosis and features of metabolic syndrome in obese Zucker fa/fa rats.* Hepatology (Baltimore, Md. 2007 Jul;46(1):122-9.

[126] Zuhri-Yafi MI, Brosnan PG, Hardin DS. *Treatment of type 2 diabetes mellitus in children and adolescents.* J Pediatr Endocrinol Metab. 2002 Apr;15 Suppl 1:541-6.

[127] Freemark M, Bursey D. *The effects of metformin on body mass index and glucose tolerance in obese adolescents with fasting hyperinsulinemia and a family history of type 2 diabetes.* Pediatrics. 2001 Apr;107(4):E55.

[128] Kay JP, Alemzadeh R, Langley G, D'Angelo L, Smith P, Holshouser S. *Beneficial effects of metformin in normoglycemic morbidly obese adolescents.* Metabolism: clinical and experimental. 2001 Dec;50(12):1457-61.

[129] Bugianesi E, Gentilcore E, Manini R, Natale S, Vanni E, Villanova N, et al. *A randomized controlled trial of metformin versus vitamin E or prescriptive diet in nonalcoholic fatty liver disease.* The American journal of gastroenterology. 2005 May;100(5):1082-90.

[130] Nair S, Diehl AM, Wiseman M, Farr GH, Jr., Perrillo RP. *Metformin in the treatment of non-alcoholic steatohepatitis: a pilot open label trial.* Alimentary pharmacology and therapeutics. 2004 Jul 1;20(1):23-8.

[131] Tock L, Damaso AR, de Piano A, Carnier J, Sanches PL, Lederman HM, et al. *Long-term effects of metformin and lifestyle modification on nonalcoholic Fatty liver disease obese adolescents.* Journal of obesity.2010.

[132] Lavine JE, Schwimmer JB, Van Natta ML, Molleston JP, Murray KF, Rosenthal P, et al. *Effect of vitamin E or metformin for treatment of nonalcoholic fatty liver disease in children and adolescents: the TONIC randomized controlled trial.* Jama. Apr 27;305(16):1659-68.

[133] Fu JF, Liang L, Zou CC, Hong F, Wang CL, Wang XM, et al. *Prevalence of the metabolic syndrome in Zhejiang Chinese obese children and adolescents and the effect of metformin combined with lifestyle intervention.* International journal of obesity (2005). 2007 Jan;31(1):15-22.

[134] Yu JG, Javorschi S, Hevener AL, Kruszynska YT, Norman RA, Sinha M, et al. *The effect of thiazolidinediones on plasma adiponectin levels in normal, obese, and type 2 diabetic subjects.* Diabetes. 2002 Oct;51(10):2968-74.

[135] Shimizu H, Tsuchiya T, Sato N, Shimomura Y, Kobayashi I, Mori M. *Troglitazone reduces plasma leptin concentration but increases hunger in NIDDM patients.* Diabetes care. 1998 Sep;21(9):1470-4.

[136] Neuschwander-Tetri BA, Brunt EM, Wehmeier KR, Oliver D, Bacon BR. *Improved nonalcoholic steatohepatitis after 48 weeks of treatment with the PPAR-gamma ligand rosiglitazone.* Hepatology (Baltimore, Md. 2003 Oct;38(4):1008-17.

[137] Ratziu V, Giral P, Jacqueminet S, Charlotte F, Hartemann-Heurtier A, Serfaty L, et al. *Rosiglitazone for nonalcoholic steatohepatitis: one-year results of the randomized placebo-controlled Fatty Liver Improvement with Rosiglitazone Therapy (FLIRT) Trial.* Gastroenterology. 2008 Jul;135(1):100-10.

[138] Nathan DM. *Rosiglitazone and cardiotoxicity--weighing the evidence.* The New England journal of medicine. 2007 Jul 5;357(1):64-6.

[139] Lavine JE. *Vitamin E treatment of nonalcoholic steatohepatitis in children: a pilot study.* The Journal of pediatrics. 2000 Jun;136(6):734-8.

[140] Vajro P, Mandato C, Franzese A, Ciccimarra E, Lucariello S, Savoia M, et al. *Vitamin E treatment in pediatric obesity-related liver disease: a randomized study.* Journal of pediatric gastroenterology and nutrition. 2004 Jan;38(1):48-55.

[141] Laurin J, Lindor KD, Crippin JS, Gossard A, Gores GJ, Ludwig J, et al. *Ursodeoxycholic acid or clofibrate in the treatment of non-alcohol-induced steatohepatitis: a pilot study.* Hepatology (Baltimore, Md. 1996 Jun;23(6):1464-7.

[142] Lindor KD, Kowdley KV, Heathcote EJ, Harrison ME, Jorgensen R, Angulo P, et al. *Ursodeoxycholic acid for treatment of nonalcoholic steatohepatitis: results of a randomized trial.* Hepatology (Baltimore, Md. 2004 Mar;39(3):770-8.

[143] Dixon JB, Bhathal PS, Hughes NR, O'Brien PE. *Nonalcoholic fatty liver disease: Improvement in liver histological analysis with weight loss.* Hepatology (Baltimore, Md. 2004 Jun;39(6):1647-54.

[144] Inge TH, Krebs NF, Garcia VF, Skelton JA, Guice KS, Strauss RS, et al. *Bariatric surgery for severely overweight adolescents: concerns and recommendations.* Pediatrics. 2004 Jul;114(1):217-23.

[145] Apovian CM, Baker C, Ludwig DS, Hoppin AG, Hsu G, Lenders C, et al. *Best practice guidelines in pediatric/adolescent weight loss surgery.* Obesity research. 2005 Feb;13(2):274-82.

[146] Keidar A, Hecht L, Weiss R. *Bariatric surgery in obese adolescents. Current opinion in clinical nutrition and metabolic care.* May;14(3):286-90.

[147] O'Brien PE, Sawyer SM, Laurie C, Brown WA, Skinner S, Veit F, et al. *Laparoscopic adjustable gastric banding in severely obese adolescents: a randomized trial.* Jama. Feb 10;303(6):519-26.

[148] Mattar SG, Velcu LM, Rabinovitz M, Demetris AJ, Krasinskas AM, *Barinas-Mitchell E, et al. Surgically-induced weight loss significantly*

improves nonalcoholic fatty liver disease and the metabolic syndrome. Annals of surgery. 2005 Oct;242(4):610-7; discussion 8-20.

[149] Barker KB, Palekar NA, Bowers SP, Goldberg JE, Pulcini JP, Harrison SA. *Non-alcoholic steatohepatitis: effect of Roux-en-Y gastric bypass surgery.* The American journal of gastroenterology. 2006 Feb;101(2):368-73.

[150] Yalamanchili K, Saadeh S, Klintmalm GB, Jennings LW, Davis GL. *Nonalcoholic fatty liver disease after liver transplantation for cryptogenic cirrhosis or nonalcoholic fatty liver disease.* Liver Transpl. Apr;16(4):431-9.

[151] Manco M, Bottazzo G, DeVito R, Marcellini M, Mingrone G, Nobili V. *Nonalcoholic fatty liver disease in children.* Journal of the American College of Nutrition. 2008 Dec;27(6):667-76.

In: Liver Disease and Peritonitis
Editor: Mao Kang Voung et al.

ISBN 978-1-61942-080-9

Chapter 3

Peritonitis in Cirrhosis: Pathogenesis, Diagnosis and Therapy

Claudia Cesaro**, *Angelo Tiso and Carmelina Loguercio

Department of Clinical and Experimental Internistica
"F. Magrassi and A. Lanzara", Gastroenterology Unit,
Second University of Naples, Naples, Italy

Abstract

Cirrhosis is the end stage liver disease and there are many complications occurring in the course of this disease. Bacterial infections are an important complication of cirrhosis and account for significant morbidity and mortality.

Spontaneous bacterial peritonitis (SBP) is the most common infection in cirrhosis, accounting for 25% of infections and occurs when ascites is infected; the word spontaneous indicates that infection of ascitic fluid occurs in absence of an identified intra-abdominal source of infection, unlike other form of peritonitis.

---

* Corresponding author: Tel. : +393335225472; E-mail address: cesaro.claudia@libero.it Via Pansini n.5 80131 Naples, Italy

The pathogenetic mechanism of SBP is a condition known as bacterial translocation (BT) defined as a migration of bacteria or their products from the gut to mesenteric lymph nodes or to other organs. In fact most of SBP is caused by Gram-negative bacteria (GNB) of intestinal origin.

Through an early diagnosis and treatment, the mortality of SPB was reduced to 20%.

An empirical antibiotic therapy should be initiated immediately upon diagnosis, taking into account that the main causative agents of the SBP are GNB aerobic bacteria and an antibiotic prophylaxis should be performed in any patient at risk (eg patients with digestive bleeding, patients with a previously history of SBP).

This review summarizes the main knowledge about peritonitis in cirrhosis, from pathogenesis to therapy.

Introduction

Bacterial infections are an important complication of cirrhosis and account for significant mortality and morbidity particularly in hospitalized patients; bacterial infections occur in 32-34% of this kind of patients and in 45% of patients admitted with gastrointestinal haemorrhage [1-4]. The most frequent of bacterial infections in cirrhosis is spontaneous bacterial peritonitis (SBP) [3] defined as an infection of ascites that occurs in absence of contiguous sources of infection (e.g. intestinal perforation, intra-abdominal abscess) and in absence of an intra-abdominal inflammatory focus such as an abscess, acute pancreatitis or cholecystitis [5].

In 1964 Conn first used the term "spontaneous bacterial peritonitis", describing six episodes of SBP in five cirrhotic patients [6] although the first descriptions of this disease appeared as early as in 1907 and the years between this date and 1958 in French and German literature [7-10], while the first reports in the English literature were those of Kerr in 1963 [11] and Conn in 1964 [6].

Since Conn's paper, reports regarding SBP have been growing dramatically in subsequent years, but in the past this condition, causing deterioration of patients with cirrhosis with a reported mortality of 90%, was underdiagnosed and undertreated, leading to now avoidable deaths, but at the time viewed as inexplicable and mysterious [12]. Nowadays data of prevalence (>20% on admission to the hospital, prior to the era of prevention, with half the episodes present at the time of admission and the remainder acquired during hospitalization [13,14]) allow to consider this complication quite common [15]. Today SBP is a treatable and preventable condition; this improvement in diagnosis and treatment is due to better knowledge about diagnostic criteria and the pathophysiological mechanisms of this disease. However despite this improvement, the incidence of SBP in cirrhotics with ascites ranges from 7% to 30 % per annum [16,17] and the hospital mortality rate is approximately 32% [18].

Pathogenesis

The infection of ascitic fluid determining the onset of peritonitis in cirrhosis is defined "spontaneous" because it occurs in absence of contiguous sources of infection, as it happens instead, in other forms of peritonitis. However the genesis of this kind of peritonitis has been well clarified in recent years, so authors suggested that we should now drop the word ''spontaneous'[12]. Moreover beside the so-called "spontaneous" forms of peritonitis, some reports have also signalled the possibility of abdominal paracentesis-induced SBP with a very high incidence in an era prior to disinfection and safety measures [19]. Notwithstanding this recent studies have established the safety profile of abdominal paracentesis [20].

Spontaneous peritonitis in cirrhosis is supported by a condition known as bacterial translocation (BT) defined as a migration of bacteria or their products from the gut to mesenteric lymph nodes or to other organs [21, 22]. It is therefore clear that the microorganisms more commonly involved in SBP come from the gut: *Escherichia coli* (70%), *Klebsiella* species (10%), *Proteus* species, *Enterococcus faecalis* (4% each), *Pseudomonas* species (2%) and others (6%) [23]. Translocation of bacteria and bacterial endotoxin, particularly LPS (bacterial lipopolysaccharide from Gram-negative bacteria) is a key mechanism that generally determines also the progression of liver damage; in fact LPS levels are directly connected with the severity of liver disease, and it is among the causes giving rise to a complex series of interrelated events that lead to the development of cirrhosis and its complications including SBP [24, 25].

BT may occur as a consequence of bacterial overgrowth, immune dysfunction and altered intestinal permeability [26].

A small intestinal bacterial overgrowth (SIBO), defined as $>10^5$ total colony-forming units/ml jejunal secretions, frequently occurs in cirrhosis with a prevalence ranging from 48% to 73% and is usually associated with endotoxemia [27, 28]. Patients with SBP have a higher prevalence of SIBO compared to those without SBP; on the contrary, patients with SIBO have a higher incidence of SBP compared to those who do not have a large bacterial overgrowth. These findings further stress the close relationship between intestinal bacteria and liver disease–related complications [29, 30]

This condition seems to be mainly the result of two mechanisms: acid-suppressive therapy [31, 32] and an intestinal hypo-dysmotility, the latter still having an unknown basic mechanism [33, 34]. Moreover SIBO seems directly related to the vascular abnormalities in the splanchnic area; in fact in a more recent study, an anomalous propagation of peristaltic waves has been found in patients with portal hypertension compared with those without portal hypertension [35].

As regards immune dysfunction, in presence of cirrhosis there are several abnormalities of both the systemic and local immune systems leading to a decrease in ability to clear cytokines, bacteria, and endotoxins from circulation. The reticular endotelium system (RES), with Kupffer cells and sinusoidal endothelial cells representing the main component of the RES, is the major defence mechanism against infections and bacteremia, able to clear bacteria [36]. However, the activities of RES are decreased in cirrhosis [37]; in fact porto-systemic shunts, moving away blood from the liver, prevent liver from clearing bacteria and endotoxin from circulation [38].

Moreover in rats with experimentally induced cirrhosis there is a marked decrease of IFNγ leading to damage to the phagocytic activity of macrophages and to other cells, significantly reducing bacterial phagocytosis and bacterial killing [39].

Finally a great deal of evidence indicates that patients with cirrhosis could present increased intestinal permeability related to the presence of portal hypertension with consequent hypertensive enteropathy and related to a lipid peroxidation of the brush border membrane due to a condition of altered oxide-reductive state [40-42].

Hence the above reported conditions favor the escape of intestinal bacteria into the blood causing a prolonged bacteremia, and later, the invasion of ascitic fluid determining the onset of peritonitis. Afterwards starting from SBP, as well as from any other bacterial infection in cirrhosis, the enhanced production of pro-inflammatory cytokines and other toxic metabolites can lead to the onset and propagation of a systemic inflammatory state. This state, in its turn, may induce vascular and coagulative alterations until the development of SIRS (systemic inflammatory response syndrome) that along with vascular alterations of cirrhosis, can induce shock and death [43, 44].

Factors associated with greater risk for SBP are a severely decompensated cirrhosis (high Child Pugh class), gastrointestinal bleeding, renal failure, low ascitic fluid protein concentration [45]. Particularly a recent report has demonstrated that renal dysfunction is the most important independent predictor of mortality in cirrhotic patients [46]. Moreover patients who have already had an episode of SBP are at increased risk of presenting a new episode. It is estimated that within 1 year 50–70% of patients surviving the first episode of SBP will develop further episodes [22].

Clinical Manifestations of SBP and Diagnosis

Clinical manifestation of SBP ranges from a lack of symptoms (thirteen percent [47], particularly in outpatients) to fever, abdominal pain, abdominal tenderness, worsening of liver function, gastrointestinal bleeding; in severe cases, especially when SBP is complicated with sepsis, clinical picture may occur with altered mental status or encephalopathy, vomiting, ileus, reduced urine output or hemodynamics instability [1]. In this case, the diagnosis of sepsis can be difficult because some clinical features of cirrhosis such as hypersplenism, high basal heart rate, hyperventilation due to hepatic encephalopathy or increase in body temperature, can mask the presence of sepsis [44]. The increase in body temperature greater than 37.8 °C, the presence of abdominal pain, continuous type, different from tense ascites, an altered mental status generally should always be investigated, when suspecting SBP [19].

In presence of all the conditions mentioned above, a diagnostic paracentesis is recommended [48]. and it should be performed in all cirrhotic patients with ascites on hospital admission, even for reasons other than ascites, in patients with ascites and gastrointestinal haemorrhage before the administration of prophylactic antibiotics and in patients with any signs of systemic inflammation [49].

As mentioned above, the paracentesis is now considered a safe procedure with a very low incidence of complications, especially if the procedure is preceded by correction of coagulopathy (a clinically evident hyperfibrinolysis or disseminated intravascular coagulation contraindicate paracentesis [50]), if present, and if it is practiced with trans-abdominal ultrasound assistance; the main complications [51] include bleeding (hemoperitoneum or abdominal wall hematoma), visceral perforation, local infection at the site of paracentesis, or peritonitis. The most common complication is ascitic fluid leak post paracentesis avoidable by keeping the patient in the right side position for a few hours.

Once the ascitic fluid is removed, it is necessary to practice the cell analysis and culture to diagnose SBP. [52].

Ascitic Fluid Cell Analysis

Practical guidelines and experts' consensus reports suggest that diagnosis of SBP is based on polymorphonuclear leukocytes (PMNL) count in ascitic fluid. In fact peritoneal infection causes an inflammatory reaction resulting in an increased number of PMN. In the past a fluid PMNL count >500/mm^3 (ml) combined with a value of pH ≤7.34 or a blood–ascitic fluid gradient >0.10, was considered accurate for diagnosis [53].

Instead today only the PMNL count is considered satisfactory with a greatest sensitivity reached with a PMNL count of 250/mm^3 (ml), although the greatest specificity is reached with a cut off of 500 PMN/mm^3[16, 44, 54]. If the tap is traumatic or if patients have an hemorrhagic ascites (RBC count >10000/mm^3) the PMN count should be corrected, subtracting from the measured PMN count, 1 PMN for every 250 red cells [47]. A PMN count of more than 250/mm^3 constitutes an indication to empirically initiate antibiotic treatment as evidence of a local inflammatory reaction, since ascites culture is negative in approximately 40% of patients [55].

PMN cell count is routinely performed with a light microscope in a manual counting chambre: after centrifuging ascitic fluid, nine millilitres of the supernatant are discharged and 40 μL of the remaining fluid are diluted with 800 μL of Turk's fluid and used to fill the counting chamber. Another 10 mL sample of ascitic fluid is stained with Giemsa for the PMN percentage determination. Using this procedure the results are available many hours post-paracentesis or sometimes even the next day exposing patients to a higher risk of death, the SBP being a life-threatening condition [56].

This has pushed researchers to look for alternative means for a rapid diagnosis e.g. automated cell counters or reagent strips (commonly used as urine Dipsticks).

Recent studies suggest that automated counting is equally efficient and may replace manual counts [57, 58], and few peer reviewed studies support a routine use of reagent strips in clinical practice [59-61], although a critical review of 19 studies has shown a low sensivity of reagent strips and a high risk of false negative results [62]. In conclusion there are no sufficient data to recommend use of automates cell counting or reagent strips for a rapid diagnosis of SBP [48].

Ascitic Fluid Culture

Ascitic fluid culture is performed using blood culture bottle with a minimum account of fluid for each bottle of 10 ml [49]. Ascitic fluid culture is not necessary for diagnosis of SBP since it is frequentely negative, but it is recommended in antibiotic therapy [48].

Cultures are positive in less than 40% of cases and the epidemiology of ascites bacterial infections differs depending on whether the infection is nosocomial (with a predominance of Gram positive bacteria) or community acquired (with a predominante of Gram negative) [63, 44, 64].

Practical guidelines suggest that blood cultures should be also performed in patients with increased ascitic fluid PMN count or in patients with suspected SBP before initiating antibiotic administration [48].

SBP Variants

Variants of SBP are bacterascites (monomicrobial non-neutrocytic bacterascites) and culture negative neutrocytic ascites (CNNA).

Bacteriascites occurs when patients have a PMNL count $<250/mm^3$ with a positive ascitic fluid culture; this happens when bacteria colonize ascitic fluid without causing inflammatory reaction or colonize ascites from a concomitant extraperitoneal infection (e.g. pneumonia or urinary tract infection) . It can be also the first step in the development of SBP.

The management is the follow: patients should be treated with antibiotics if they show signs of systemic inflammation or infections or if they have a PMNL count $>250/mm^3$ in a second sample (a second tap is recommended after three days after initial paracentesis) or a PMNL count $<250/mm^3$ with a second set of cultures positive. Patients who have for the second time a PMNL count $<250/mm^3$ with a second set of cultures negative should be only followed up [48, 49].

Culture negative neutrocytic ascites (CNNA) is the term used to describe the condition of increased PMN count in ascites and negative culture [65].

Patients with CNNA must be treated as if they had SBP, since this condition represents the expected 20% fail rate of culture to isolate the microorganisms [47].

Finally, it is important to differentiate the classical SBP from secondary peritonitis which may occur in cirrhosis and may be due to perforation or inflammation of an intra-abdominal organ. It should be suspected when there are localized abdominal signs and symptoms, when the cultures of ascites are positive for multiple microrganisms with a very high neutrophil count (particularly when the growth of anaerobic bacteria or fungi is observed), when there is an inadequate response to therapy (lack of a significant decrease or even an increase in ascitic fluid PMN cell count) or when glucose levels are <50 mg/dl or protein concentration >10 g/l or lactic dehydrogenase concentration >normal serum levels [66, 67]. When there is a strong suspicion of secondary peritonitis an appropriate radiological investigation is recommended [68].

Therapy of Spontaneous Bacterial Peritonitis

As soon as diagnosis of SBP is made (based on the PMN count), an empirical antibiotic therapy must be started without awaiting results of ascitic fluid culture [49]. Since the most common etiologic agents are Escherichia coli, Klebsiella, Staphylococcus aureus, Enterococcus faecalis, Streptococcus pneumonia and other streptococcal and enterococcal species, the recommended antibiotics are third generation cephalosporins as they cover most causative organisms and have a good safety profile [69]. Cefotaxime is the most commonly used antibiotic of this class because it reaches high concentrations in ascites during treatment; a dose of 4gr/day and one of 8gr/day are equally effective as well as a 5-day and a 10-day therapy; therefore the short-term course is recommended [70-72]. The use of other cephalosporins, including cefonicid, ceftriaxone, ceftizoxime and ceftazidime produces similar results as concerns SBP resolution, if compared to cefotaxime [73, 74]. Alternative options are ofloxacin [75], ciprofloxacin [76] and amoxycillin/clavulanic acid [77] while aminoglycosides should be avoided as initial empirical antibiotic therapy. Patients with SBP receiving prophylaxis with quinolones or patients living in areas with a high prevalence of quinolone-resistant bacteria, should not be treated with this kind of antibiotics;

in these patients cefotaxime administration seems to be the most adequate antibiotic regimen [49].

After 2 days of antibiotic therapy one follow-up paracentesis is recommended to guide the effect of treatment by determining the PMN count in ascitic fluid. When a decrease of ascitic neutrophil count in ascitic fluid occur and cultures become sterile if positive at diagnosis, we can think that SBP is clearing up (this happens in 90% of patients). A treatment failure should be suspected when there is a deterioration of the condition of the patients within the first hours of antibiotic therapy or when no significant reduction in ascitic PMN count of less than 25% compared to levels at diagnosis is observed. In case of treatment failure a secondary bacterial peritonitis must be excluded and antibiotic therapy should be rapidly modifying according to the *in vitro* susceptibility of isolated bacteria in patients with culture-positive SBP or empirically in patients with culture-negative SBP [48, 49]. Moreover EASL practice guidelines recommend to treat SBP with intravenous albumin since a hepatorenal syndrome (HRS) occurs in 30% of patients treated with antibiotics alone. Some reports show that albumin (1,5 gr/kg at diagnosis and 1gr/kg on day 3) improves survival, decreasing the frequency of HRS [48].

Prophylaxis of Spontaneous Bacterial Peritonitis

Practical guidelines recommend prophylactic antibiotic therapy for SBP in high-risk patients because it reduces the incidence of the first episode (primary prophylaxis), and the recurrence rate (secondary prophylaxis) [78, 79].

Given the high cost and the risk of bacterial resistance, only three high-risk patient populations have been identified: patients with acute gastrointestinal haemorrhage; patients with low ascitic fluid protein concentration and no prior history of SBP (primary prophylaxis); patients with a previous history of SBP (secondary prophylaxis).

Cirrhotic Patients with Gastrointestinal Haemorrhage

Bacterial infections (including SBP), occuring between 25% and 56% of patients with gastrointestinal bleeding, are associated with an increased rate of failure to control bleeding and rebleeding [80-82]. Moreover they represent the most important mortality risk together with hepatic functional status (assessed by Child- Pugh score) and renal dysfunction (assessed by creatinine serum levels) [83]. Consequently treatment of variceal gastrointestinal bleeding includes short-term antibiotic prophylaxis in addition to volume expansion, haemorrhage control and use of vasoconstrictors [84].

Evidence suggests that antibiotic prophylaxis prevents infection in gastrointestinal bleeding, decreases risk of rebleeding and the incidence of mortality [44, 63, 85, 86].

Several groups of antibiotics such as quinolones, cephalosporins or aminoglycosides have been assessed [4], but recommended drugs are mainly oral quinolones (norfloxacin 400 mg/12h for 7 days) or intravenous cephalosporins (ceftriaxone 1 g/day for 7 days) [84, 49]. According to a recent report demonstrating that ceftriaxone is more effective than norfloxacin in the prevention of infections in patients with gastrointestinal bleeding and advanced cirrhosis, EASL clinical practice guidelines recommend ceftriaxone as antibiotic of choice in patients with gastrointestinal bleeding and severe liver disease and oral norfloxacin or an alternative oral quinolone in patients with less severe liver disease [48].

Despite this, in a recent Cochrane review evaluating seventeen trials (including a total of 1891 cirrhotic patients with upper gastrointestinal bleeding) authors conclude that benefits of prophylactic therapy are observed independently of the antibiotic assessed; therefore no specific antibiotic regimen can be recommended more than another. Thus, antibiotic selection should be made considering local conditions such as bacterial resistance profile and treatment cost [85].

Patients with Low Ascitic Fluid Protein Concentration and No Prior History of SBP

There are insufficient data on the efficacy of quinolones in preventing SBP or in improving survival in patients with moderate liver disease and ascites protein concentration lower than 15gr/L, while one double-blind placebo controlled randomized trial has shown that norfloxacin (400 mg/day) reduces risk of SBP in patients with severe liver disease and ascitic fluid protein concentration lower than 15gr/L, so EASL clinical practice guidelines suggest that these patients should be trated with a long-term prophylaxis with norfloxacin [48].

Patients with a Previous History of SBP

Within 1 year 50–70% of patients surviving the first episode of SBP will develop further episodes [22] with a probability of survival at 1 year after episode of 30-50%. Several studies have investigated the effectiveness of different antibiotics (norfloxacin, ciprofloxacin, trimethoprim-sulfamethoxazole) in secondary prophylaxis [87-89]. According to studies results long-term antibiotic administration is advised for all patients surviving the first episode of SBP with norfloxacin as treatment of choice (400 mg/day orally); alternative antibiotics are ciprofloxacin (750 mg once weekly orally) and co-trimoxazole (800 mg sulfamethoxazole and 160 mg trimethoprim daily orally) with a less strong evidence than norfloxacin [48]. Instead it is still unclear if treatment could be continued until liver transplantation or death and discontinued in the case of a improvement of liver disease [49]. Anyhow patients recovering from SBP should be considered for liver transplantation since survival expectancy after liver transplantation is currently much higher [90, 91].

References

[1] Tandon P, Garcia-Tsao G. Bacterial Infections, Sepsis, and Multiorgan Failure in Cirrhosis. *Seminars in liver disease* 2008;28:26-42.

[2] Borzio M, Salerno F, Piantoni L, Cazzaniga M, Angeli P, Bissoli F, Boccia S, Colloredo-Mels G, Corigliano P, Fornaciari G, Marenco G, Pistarà R, Salvagnini M, Sangiovanni A. Bacterial infection in patients with advanced cirrhosis: a multicentre prospective study. *Dig Liver Dis* 2001;33:41–48.

[3] Fernandez J, Navasa M, Gómez J, Colmenero J, Vila J, Arroyo V, Rodés J. Bacterial infections in cirrhosis: epidemiological changes with invasive procedures and norfloxacin prophylaxis. *Hepatology* 2002;35: 140–148.

[4] Bernard B, Grange JD, Khac EN, Amiot X, Opolon P, Poynard T. Antibiotic prophylaxis for the prevention of bacterial infections in cirrhotic patients with gastrointestinal bleeding: a meta-analysis. *Hepatology* 1999;29:1655–1661.

[5] Garcia-Tsao G. Spontaneous bacterial peritonitis: a historical perspective. *J Hepatol* 2004; 41: 522-527.

[6] Conn HO. Spontaneous peritonitis and bacteremia in laennec's cirrhosis caused by enteric organisms. A relatively common but rarely recognized syndrome. *Ann. Intern. Med.* 1964; 60: 568-580.

[7] Krencker E. Bacterium coli commune als Sepsiserrenger in 2 fallen von abdominaler Krankungen. *Munchen Med .Wschr*. 1907; 54: 2095.

[8] Brule M, Hillemand P, Goutner B. Septicemie a colibacille et peritonite terminale chez une cirrhotique. *Bull. Soc. Med. Hop. Paris* 1939; 63: 1167.

[9] Cachin M. Sur un syndrome ictero-ascitique avec colibacillemie. *Rev. Med. Chir. Mal. Foie* 1955; 30:5.

[10] Caroli J, Platteborse R. Septicemie porto-cave. Cirrhosis du foie et septicemie a colibacille. *Sem. Hop. Paris* 1958; 34:112-127.

[11] Kerr DNS, Pearson DT, Read AE. Infection of ascitic fluid in patients with hepatic cirrhosis. *Gut* 1963; 4:394-398.

[12] Runyon BA. Early events in spontaneous bacterial peritonitis. *Gut* 2004; 53: 782-4.

[13] Toledo C, Salmeron JM, Rimola A, Navasa M, Arroyo V, Llach J, Ginès A, Ginès P, Rodés J. Spontaneous bacterial peritonitis in cirrhosis: predictive factors of infection resolution and survival in patients treated with cefotaxime. *Hepatology* 1993; 17: 251-7.

[14] Llovet JM, Planas R, Morillas R, Quer JC, Cabré E, Boix J, Humbert P, Guilera M, Doménech E, Bertrán X, et al.. Short-term prognosis of cirrhotics with spontaneous bacterial peritonitis: multivariate study. *Am. J. Gastroenterol* 1993; 88: 388-92

[15] Pinzello G, Simonetti RG, Craxi A Di Piazza S, Spanò C, Pagliaro L. Spontaneous bacterial peritonitis: a prospective investigation in predominantly nonalcoholic cirrhotic patients. *Hepatology* 1983;3:545-9.

[16] Rimola A, Garcia-Tsao G, Navasa M, Piddock LJ, Planas R, Bernard B, Inadomi JM.Diagnosis, treatment and prophylaxis of spontaneous bacterial peritonitis: a consensus document. *J. Hepatol.* 2000;32:142–53.

[17] Sapey T, Kabissa D, Fort E, Laurin C, Mendler MH. Instant diagnosis of spontaneous bacterial peritonitis using leukocyte esterase reagent strips: Nephur-TestH vs. MultistixSGH. *Liver Int* 2005;25:343–8.

[18] Thuluvath PJ, Morss S, Thompson R. Spontaneous bacterial peritonitis--in-hospital mortality, predictors of survival, and health care costs from 1988 to 1998. *Am. J. Gastroenterol.* 2001;96:1232–1236.

[19] Koulaouzidis A, Bhat S, Saeed AA. Spontaneous bacterial peritonitis. *World J Gastroenterol*. 2009 Mar 7;15(9):1042-9. Review.

[20] Runyon BA. Paracentesis of ascitic fluid: a safe procedure. *Arch. Intern. Med.* 1986;146:2259–61.

[21] Wiest R, Rath HC. Gastrointestinal disorders of the critically ill. Bacterial translocation in the gut. *Best Pract. Res. Clin. Gastroenterol.* 2003;17:397-425.

[22] Berg RD, Garlington AW. Translocation of certain indigenous bacteria from the gastrointestinal tract to the mesenteric lymph nodes and other organs in a gnotobiotic mouse model. *Infect. Immun.* 1979;23:403-11.

[23] Arroyo V, Bataller R, Gine`s P. *Spontaneous Bacterial Peritonitis*, eds. O'Grady and Lake's comprehensive clinical hepatology, 1st ed. Barcelona: Mosby, 2000:7.10–7.14.

[24] Lin RS, Lee FY, Lee SD, Tsai YT, Lin HC, Lu RH, Hsu WC, Huang CC, Wang SS, Lo KJ. Endotoxemia in patients with chronic liver diseases: relationship to severity of liver diseases, presences of esophageal varices, and hyperdynamic circulation. *J. Hepatol.* 1995;22:165-72.

[25] Bigatello LM, Broitman SA, Fattori L, Di Paoli M, Pontello M, Bevilacqua G, Nespoli A. Endotoxemia, encephalopathy, and mortality in cirrhotic patients. *Am. J. Gastroenterol.* 1987;82:11-5.

[26] Riordan SM, Williams R. The intestinal flora and bacterial infection in cirrhosis. *J. Hepatol.* 2006;45:744-7.

[27] Yang CY, Chang CS, Chen GH. Small intestinal bacterial overgrowth in patients with liver cirrhosis, diagnosed with glucose H2 or CH4 breath tests. *Scand. J. Gastroenterol.* 1998;33:867-71.

[28] Bauer TM, Schwacha H, Steinbruckner B, Brinkmann FE, Ditzen AK, Aponte JJ, Pelz K, Berger D, Kist M, Blum HE. Small intestinal bacterial overgrowth in human cirrhosis is associated with systemic endotoxaemia. *Am. J. Gastroenterol.* 2002;97:2364-70.

[29] Morencos FC, de las Heras-Castano G, Martin-Ramos L, López Arias MJ, Ledesma F, Pons Romero F. Small bowel bacterial overgrowth in patients with alcoholic cirrhosis. *Dig. Dis. Sci.* 1995;40:1252-6.

[30] Bauer TM, Steinbruckner B, Brinkmann FE, Ditzen AK, Schwacha H, Aponte JJ, Pelz K, Kist M, Blum HE. Small intestinal bacterial overgrowth in patients with cirrhosis: prevalence and relation with spontaneous bacterial peritonitis. *Am. J. Gastroenterol.* 2001;96:2962-7.

[31] Shindo K, Machida M, Miyakawa K, Fukumura M. A syndrome of cirrhosis, achlorhydria, small intestinal bacterial overgrowth, and fat malabsorption. *Am. J. Gastroenterol.* 1993;88:2084–91.

[32] Bauer TM, Schwacha H, Steinbru¨ckner B, Brinkmann FE, Ditzen AK, Kist M, Blum HE. Diagnosis of small intestinal bacterial overgrowth in patients with cirrhosis of the liver: Poor performance of the glucose breath hydrogen test. *J. Hepatol.* 2000;32:382–6.

[33] Madrid AM, Cumsille F, Defilippi C. Altered small bowel motility in patients with liver cirrhosis depends on severity of liver disease. *Dig. Dis. Sci.* 1997;42:738-42.

[34] Madrid AM, Brahm J, Buckel E, Silva G, Defilippi C. Orthotopic liver transplantation improves small bowel motility disorders in cirrhotic patients. *Am. J. Gastroenterol.* 1997;92:1044-5.

[35] Gunnarsdottir SA, Sadik R, Shev S, Simrén M, Sjövall H, Stotzer PO, Abrahamsson H, Olsson R, Björnsson ES. Small intestinal motility disturbances and bacterial overgrowth in patients with liver cirrhosis and portal hypertension. *Am. J. Gastroenterol.* 2003;98:1362-70.

[36] Bonnel AR, Bunchorntavakul C, Reddy KR. Immune Dysfunction and Infections in Patients with Cirrhosis. *Clin. Gastroenterol. Hepatol.* 2011. [Epub ahead of print]

[37] Rimola A, Soto R, Bory F, Arroyo V, Piera C, Rodes J. Reticuloendothelial system phagocytic activity in cirrhosis and its relation to bacterial infections and prognosis. *J. Hepatol.* 1984;4:53-8.

[38] Ghassemi S, Garcia-Tsao G. Prevention and treatment of infections in patients with cirrhosis. *Best Pract. Res. Clin. Gastroenterol* 2007;21:77–93.

[39] Inamura T, Miura S, Tsuzuki Y, Hara Y, Hokari R, Ogawa T, Teramoto K, Watanabe C, Kobayashi H, Nagata H, Ishii H. Alteration of intestinal intraepithelial lymphocytes and increased bacterial translocation in a murine model of cirrhosis. *Immunol. Lett.* 2003;90:3-11.

[40] Wiest R, Garcia-Tsao G. Bacterial translocation (BT) in cirrhosis. *Hepatology* 2005;41:422-33.

[41] Misra V, Misra SP, Dwivedi M, Gupta SC. Histomorphometric study of portal hypertensive enteropathy. *Am. J. Clin. Pathol.* 1997;108:652-7.

[42] Ramachandran A, Prabhu R, Thomas S, Reddy JB, Pulimood A, Balasubramanian KA. Intestinal mucosal alterations in experimental cirrhosis in the rat: role of oxygen free radicals. *Hepatology* 2002;35:622-9.

[43] Alberti C, Brun-Buisson C, Goodman SV, Guidici D, Granton J, Moreno R, Smithies M, Thomas O, Artigas A, Le Gall JR; European Sepsis Group. Influence of systemic inflammatory response syndrome and

sepsis on outcome of critically ill infected patients. *Am. J. Respir. Crit Care Med.* 2003;168:77-84.

[44] Wong F, Bernardi M, Balk R, et al. Sepsis in cirrhosis: report on the 7th meeting of the International Ascites Club. *Gut* 2005;54:718-25.

[45] Sherlock S., Dooley J. Ascites: Sponteneous bacterial peritonitis. In Wiley-Blackwell. *Diseases of the liver and biliary system*. 2002; 132.

[46] Tandon P, Garcia-Tsao G. Renal Dysfunction Is the Most Important Independent Predictor of Mortality in Cirrhotic Patients With Spontaneous Bacterial Peritonitis. *Clinical Gastroenterology and Hepatology*. 2011;9:260–265.

[47] Runyon BA. Ascites and spontaneous bacterial peritonitis. In: Feldman M, Friedman LS, Sleisenger MH, eds. *Sleisenger and Fordran's gastrointestinal and liver disease*, 8th ed. Philadelphia: Saunders, 2006: 1935-1964.

[48] Ginès P, Angeli P, Lenz K, Møller S, Moore K, Moreau R, Merkel C, Ring-Larsen H, Bernardi M, Garcia-Tsao G, Hayers P. EASL clinical practice guidelines on the management of ascites, spontaneous bacterial peritonitis, and hepatorenal syndrome in cirrhosis. European Association for the Study of the Liver. *J. Hepatol.* 2010;53:397-417.

[49] Rimola A, García-Tsao G, Navasa M, Piddock LJ, Planas R, Bernard B, Inadomi JM. Diagnosis, treatment and prophylaxis of spontaneous bacterial peritonitis: a consensus document. International Ascites Club. *J. Hepatol.* 2000 32:142-53.

[50] Runyon BA. Management of adult patients with ascites due to cirrhosis: an update. *Hepatology* 2009; 49: 2087-2107.

[51] Nazeer SR, Dewbre H, Miller AH. Ultrasound-assisted paracentesis performed by emergency physicians vs the traditional technique: a prospective, randomized study. *Am. J. Emerg. Med.* 2005; 23: 363-367.

[52] McGibbon A, Chen GI, Peltekian KM, van Zanten SV. An evidence-based manual for abdominal paracentesis. *Dig. Dis. Sci.* 2007; 52: 3307-3315.

[53] Stassen WN, McCullough AJ, Bacan BR, et al. Immediate diagnostic criteria for bacterial infection of ascitic fluid- evaluation of ascitic fluid polymorphonuclear leukocyte count, pH, and lactate concentration, Alone and in combination. *Gastroenterology* 1986;90:1247–54.

[54] Garcia-Tsao G. Spontaneous bacterial peritonitis. *Gastroenterol. Clin. N Am.* 1992; 21: 257-75.

[55] Runyon BA, Canawati HN, Akriviadis EA. Optimization of ascitic fluid culture technique. *Gastroenterology* 1988; 95: 1351-5.

[56] Riggio O, Angeloni S. Ascitic fluid analysis for diagnosis and monitoring of spontaneous bacterial peritonitis. *World J. Gastroenterol.* 2009;15:3845-50.

[57] Angeloni S, Nicolini G, Merli M, Nicolao F, Pinto G, Aronne T, Attili AF, Riggio O Am J Validation of automated blood cell counter for the determination of polymorphonuclear cell count in the ascitic fluid of cirrhotic patients with or without spontaneous bacterial peritonitis. *Gastroenterol.* 2003; 98:1844-8.

[58] Cereto F, Genescà J, Segura R. Validation of automated blood cell counters for the diagnosis of spontaneous bacterial peritonitis. *Am. J. Gastroenterol.* 2004; 99: 1400.

[59] Castelote J, Lopez C, Gornals J, et al. Rapid diagnosis of SBP by the use of reagent strips. *Hepatology* 2002;37:893–6.

[60] The´venot T, Cadranel JF, Nguyen-Khac E, Tilmant L, Tiry C, Welty S, Merzoug N. Diagnosis of spontaneous bacterial peritonitis in cirrhotic patients by use of two reagent strips. *Eur. J. Gastroenterol. Hepatol.* 2004;16:579–83.

[61] Sapey T, Mena E, Fort E, Laurin C, Kabissa D, Runyon BA, Mendler MH. Rapid diagnosis of spontaneous bacterial peritonitis with leukocyte esterase reagent strips in a European and in an American center. *J. Gastroenterol. Hepatol* 2005;20:187–92.

[62] Nguyen-Khac E, Cadranel JF, Thevenot T, Nousbaum JB. Review article: the utility of reagent strips in the diagnosis of infected ascites in cirrhotic patients. *Aliment Pharmacol Ther.* 2008;28:282-8.

[63] Garcia-Tsao G. Current management of the complications of cirrhosis and portal hypertension: variceal hemorrhage, ascites, and spontaneous bacterial peritonitis. *Gastroenterology*. 2001;120:726-48.

[64] Fernández J, Navasa M, Gómez J, Colmenero J, Vila J, Arroyo V, Rodés J. Bacterial infections in cirrhosis: epidemiological changes with invasive procedures and norfloxacin prophylaxis. *Hepatology*. 2002;35:140-8.

[65] Pelletier G, Salmon D, Ink 0, Hannoun S, Attali P, Buffet C, Etienne JP. Culture-negative neutrocytic ascites: a less severe variant of spontaneous bacterial peritonitis. *J. Hepatol.* 1990; 10: 327-31.

[66] Runyon BA, Hoefs JC. Ascitic fluid analysis in the differentiation of spontaneous bacterial peritonitis from gastrointestinal tract perforation into ascitic fluid. *Hepatology* 1984; 4: 44-50.

[67] Runyon BA, Hoefs JC. Spontaneous vs. secondary bacterial peritonitis. Differentiation by response of ascitic fluid neutrophil count to antimicrobial therapy. *Arch. Intern. Med.* 1986; 146: 1563-5.

[68] Guarner C, Soriano G. Spontaneous bacterial peritonitis. *Semin Liver Dis.* 1997;17:203-17.

[69] Kuiper JJ, van Buuren HR, de Man RA. Review article: Management of ascites and associated complications in patients with cirrhosis. *Alimentary Pharmacology and Therapeutics* 2007;26 (Suppl 2):183–93.

[70] Felisart J, Rimola A, Arroyo V, Perez-Ayuso RM, Quintero E, Gines P, Rodes J. Cefotaxime is more effective than is ampicillin-tobramycin in cirrhotics with severe infections. *Hepatology.* 1985;5:457-62.

[71] Rimola A, Salmerón JM, Clemente G, Rodrigo L, Obrador A, Miranda ML, Guarner C, Planas R, Solá R, Vargas V. Two different dosages of cefotaxime in the treatment of spontaneous bacterial peritonitis in cirrhosis: results of a prospective, randomized, multicenter study. *Hepatology.* 1995;21:674-9.

[72] Runyon BA, McHutchison JG, Antillon MR, Akriviadis EA, Montano AA. Short-course versus long-course antibiotic treatment of spontaneous bacterial peritonitis. A randomized controlled study of 100 patients. *Gastroenterology.* 1991;100:1737-42.

[73] Rimola A, Titò Ll, Llach J, Salmeron JM, Marques F, Badalamenti S, et al. Efficacy of ceftizoxime in the treatment of severe bacterial infections in patients with cirrhosis. *Drug Invest* 1992; 4(suppl 1): 35-7.

[74] Gomez-Jimenez J, Ribera E, Gasser J, Artaza MA, DelValle 0, Pahissa A, Martínez-Vázquez JM. Randomized trial comparing ceftriaxone with cefonicid for treatment of spontaneous bacterial peritonitis in cirrhotic patients. *Antimicrob. Agents Chemother* 1993; 37: 1587-92.

[75] Navasa M, Follo A, Llovet JM, Clemente G, Vargas V, Rimola A, Marco F, Guarner C, Forné M, Planas R, Bañares R, Castells L, Jimenez De Anta MT, Arroyo V, Rodés J. Randomized, comparative study of oral ofloxacin versus intravenous cefotaxime in spontaneous bacterial peritonitis. *Gastroenterology.* 1996;111:1011-7.

[76] Terg R, Cobas S, Fassio E, Landeira G, Ríos B, Vasen W, Abecasis R, Ríos H, Guevara M. Oral ciprofloxacin after a short course of intravenous ciprofloxacin in the treatment of spontaneous bacterial peritonitis: results of a multicenter, randomized study. *J. Hepatol.* 2000;33:564-9.

[77] Ricart E, Soriano G, Novella MT, Ortiz J, Sàbat M, Kolle L, Sola-Vera J, Miñana J, Dedéu JM, Gómez C, Barrio JL, Guarner C. Amoxicillin-

clavulanic acid versus cefotaxime in the therapy of bacterial infections in cirrhotic patients. *J. Hepatol.* 2000;32:596-602.

[78] Soriano G, Guarner C, Teixido′ M, Such J, Barrios J, Enríquez J, Vilardell F. Selective intestinal decontamination prevents spontaneous bacterial peritonitis. *Gastroenterology*. 1991;100:477–481.

[79] Gine′s P, Rimola A, Planas R, Vargas V, Marco F, Almela M, Forné M, Miranda ML, Llach J, Salmerón JM, et al. Norfloxacin prevents spontaneous bacterial peritonitis recurrence in cirrhosis: results of a double-blind, placebo-controlled trial. *Hepatology*. 1990;12: 716–724.

[80] Goulis J, Armonis A, Patch D, Sabin C, Greenslade L, Burroughs AK. Bacterial infection is independently associated with failure to control bleeding in cirrhotic patients with gastrointestinal hemorrhage. *Hepatology*. 1998 27:1207-12.

[81] Vivas S, Rodriguez M, Palacio MA, Linares A, Alonso JL, Rodrigo L. Presence of bacterial infection in bleeding cirrhotic patients is independently associated with early mortality and failure to control bleeding. *Dig. Dis. Sci.* 2001 46:2752-7.

[82] Bernard B, Cadranel JF, Valla D, Escolano S, Jarlier V, Opolon P. Prognostic significance of bacterial infection in bleeding cirrhotic patients: a prospective study. *Gastroenterology*. 1995;108:1828-34.

[83] Augustin S, Muntaner L, Altamirano JT, Gonzalez A, Saperas E, Dot J, Abu-Suboh M, Armengol JR, Malagelada JR, Esteban R, Guardia J, Genescà J. Predicting early mortality after acute variceal hemorrhage based on classification and regression tree analysis. *Clinical Gastroenterology and Hepatology*. 2009;7:1347–54.

[84] Garcia-Tsao G, Lim J K. Management and treatment of patients with cirrhosis and portal hypertension: recommendations from the Department of Veterans Affairs Hepatitis C Resource Center Program and the National Hepatitis C Program. *American Journal of Gastroenterology* 2009;104:1802–29.

[85] Chavez-Tapia NC, Barrientos-Gutierrez T, Tellez-Avila FI, Soares-Weiser K, Uribe M. Antibiotic prophylaxis for cirrhotic patients with upper gastrointestinal bleeding. Cochrane Database Syst Rev. 2010;(9):CD002907.

[86] Bernard B, Grangé JD, Khac EN, Amiot X, Opolon P, Poynard T. Antibiotic prophylaxis for the prevention of bacterial infections in cirrhotic patients with gastrointestinal bleeding: a meta-analysis. *Hepatology*. 1999;29:1655-61.

[87] Rolachon A, Cordier L, Bacq Y, Nousbaum JB, Franza A, Paris JC, Fratte S, Bohn B, Kitmacher P, Stahl JP, et al. Ciprofloxacin and long-term prevention of spontaneous bacterial peritonitis: results of a prospective controlled trial. *Hepatology* 1995;22:1171–4.

[88] Novella M, Sola R, Soriano G, Andreu M, Gana J, Ortiz J, Coll S, Sàbat M, Vila MC, Guarner C, Vilardell F. Continuous versus inpatient prophylaxis of the first episode of spontaneous bacterial peritonitis with norfloxacin. *Hepatology* 1997;25:532–6.

[89] Gines P, Rimola A, Planas R, Vargas V, Marco F, Almela M, Forné M, Miranda ML, Llach J, Salmerón JM, et al. Norfloxacin prevents spontaneous bacterial peritonitis recurrence in cirrhosis: results of a double blind, placebo-controlled trial. *Hepatology* 1990;12:716–24.

[90] Kilpe VE, Krakahuer H, Wren RE. An analysis of liver transplant experience from 37 transplant centers as reported to Medicare. *Transplantation* 1993; 56: 55461.

[91] *European Liver Transplant Registry*. Data analysis 05/1968-06/1997. Hospital Paul Brousse, Villejuif, France.

Reviewed by

Marcello Persico Professor of Internal Medicine, Second University of Naples, Naples. Italy.

In: Liver Disease and Peritonitis
Editor: Mao Kang Voung et al.

ISBN 978-1-61942-080-9

Chapter 4

Ethnic Disparities in Liver Diseases

Nyingi Kemmer [*] ***and Guy W. Neff***
Division of Hepatology and Transplant Hepatology
Tampa General Medical Group, Florida, US

Abstract

Chronic liver disease is a major cause of morbidity and mortality among ethnic minorities. Additionally, ethnic variations exist in liver disease prevalence, clinical presentation, therapeutic outcome, access to health care and healthcare utilization. The numerous differences are inter-related and present unique challenges that contribute to the health diversity in the multiethnic populations. This review will discuss the existing literature on ethnic variations in chronic liver diseases. It will also provide better understanding of ethnic disparities in this population, and address clinical implications of this disparity where applicable.

Chronic liver disease is a common cause of morbidity and mortality in the United States today. According to the findings of recent epidemiologic studies,

[*] Corresponding Author: Nyingi Kemmer, MD, MPH, Tampa General Medical Group; 409 Bayshore Blvd. Tampa, FL 33606. Phone: 813-844-8686. Email : nkemmer@tgh.org

the most common etiology of chronic liver disease in this country are chronic hepatitis C virus (HCV) infection and nonalcoholic fatty liver disease (NAFLD). In addition, several reports have documented the rising incidence of hepatocellular carcinoma. Other common chronic liver diseases include chronic hepatitis B virus infection, alcoholic, autoimmune, and metabolic liver disease. Similar to other medical disorders, the clinical presentation, response to treatment, and prognosis of chronic liver diseases and their sequelae vary according to ethnicity. Previous reports focusing on chronic liver disease have documented ethnic healthcare disparities in patient access, delayed referrals as differences in utilization of resources at the institutional level for those with sequelae of advanced liver disease such as portal hypertension and hepatocellular carcinoma (HCC) [1-4].

There is little information on the interethnic variation in the clinical presentation and outcome of patients with acute and chronic liver disease. Practicing healthcare providers need to be cognizant of ethnic differences and therapeutic options as well as prognostic implications. This review will discuss the ethnic variations and implications of the most common liver diseases. The purpose is to provide a better understanding of ethnic disparities in liver disease, and to address clinical implications of this disparity where applicable. Due to the lack of consistency in the classification across published studies, in this review ethnicity and race will be used interchangeably. Ethnicity/race will be categorized as (i) White or Caucasian (ii) Black or African American (iii) Hispanic or Latino (iv)Asian and (v) Others.

Viral Hepatitis: HBV and HCV

Hepatitis C: Chronic HCV infection affects 170 million people world-wide. In the United States, the prevalence is two-fold higher in the black population than in the white or Mexican American population (3% compared with 1.5% and 1.3%, respectively) [5]. To date, six HCV genotypes (1–6) have been identified. The significance of the HCV genotype is in relation to antiviral therapy response, with genotype 1 having the lowest response rate. In a recent population-based study, the rate of infection with genotype 1 was disproportionately higher among black individuals (90.9%) when compared to white (69.6%) and Mexican Americans (71.2%) [6]. Therefore, it is not surprising that a larger percentage of black patients have disease that is non-responsive to the currently approved antiviral drugs. The sustained virologic response (SVR) rate for black patients with genotype 1 infection is 19–28%, compared with 45– 55% for white patients. In the earlier studies, among Mexican Americans a similar reduced virologic response rate has been observed and estimated to be slightly better than in Blacks but significantly lower than in Whites [7,8]. In addition, a clinical trial specifically designed to evaluate therapeutic response in Latinos, confirmed the results of the latter studies showing a similar lower SVR in Latinos compared to non-Latino whites (34% vs 49%) [9,10]. However, in a recent study by Muir et al, the investigators report that using an individualized dosing regimen the overall SVR rates were 44% for white, 22% for African American (AA), 38% for Hispanic and 59% for Asian Americans. In this study, there was no significant difference in SVR between Hispanic and White [10]. Although patients with genotypes 2 and 3 are more responsive to antiviral therapy, a similar ethnic difference has been reported, with Blacks demonstrating lower virologic response in comparison to Caucasians [11].

Recent studies using protease inhibitors in combination with pegylated interferon and ribavirin, has shown significant improvements in SVR across ethnic groups in both naïve and previously treated HCV infected patients [12-15]. In the SPRINT-2 trial for naïve HCV patients, in which the study participants received 4 weeks of peginterferon alfa-2b and ribavirin during the lead-in period and then 44 wks of boceprevir plus peginterfeon and ribavirin, the overall SVR was 68%, with 53% for blacks and 68% for non-black [12]. In the ADVANCE trial for naïve patients, study participants received Telaprevir with peginterferon alfa-2a and ribavirin for 12 weeks followed by peginterferon alfa-2a and ribavirin alone for 12 weeks if HCV RNA was undetectable at wks 4 and 12 or for 36 weeks if HCV RNA was detectable at either time point. In the latter study, the SVR based on race was white 75% and black 62% and for ethnicity Hispanic 74% and non-hispanic 75% [13]. Though there is a significant increase in response rates for all ethnic groups, blacks consistently have lower SVR in comparison to others.

The lower response rates amongst blacks appears to be multi-factorial, with viral kinetic studies demonstrating impaired HCV inhibition in black individuals, and immunologic studies showing an ethnic variation in cytokine profiles [16,17]. Furthermore in a recent study, investigators found that a genetic polymorphism near the IL28B gene (Interferon- λ-3) the C/C genotype was significantly associated with virologic response to interferon-based therapy for patients infected with HCV genotype 1. This genetic polymorphism explains in part the observed ethnic difference in SVR across ethnic groups since the C/C genotype occurs less frequently in blacks, has intermediate frequency in Hispanics and Caucasians and is more frequent in Asians [18,19] Overall, after adjustments for predictors the chances of virologic clearance varied with IL28B polymorphisms with reports of SVR rates of 78% (C/C genotype), 38% (T/C genotype) and 26% (T/T genotype) [18]. More studies are needed to aid our understanding of the influence of the observed ethnic differences in genetic polymorphism, cytokine profile and quasispecies in patients with chronic HCV infection.

Ethnic differences in liver histology have been demonstrated in patients with chronic hepatitis C. In a recent prospective study, African American patients were found to have a significantly lower prevalence of hepatic steatosis when compared to Caucasians, while a similar study reported a higher prevalence of hepatic steatosis in Latinos compared to Caucasians (54.7 vs 43.2%) [20,21]. Despite these findings, the role of hepatic steatosis as an independent predictor of response to therapy in genotype 1-infected patients is unclear [22-24]. In addition to these ethnic differences in hepatic steatosis, African Americans have less piecemeal necrosis and necroinflammatory activity than Caucasians, resulting in an overall lower hepatic activity index score [25,26]. Differences in histologic stage of hepatitis C has also been reported across ethnic groups, with several studies documenting more advanced fibrosis in Hispanics in comparison to Blacks and Whites[26-29]. Of note, a recent study evaluating the association of BMI and ethnicity on fibrosis progression, found BMI and ethnicity to be directly associated. In the latter study, at presentation cirrhosis was present in 50%, 38% and 24% in Hispanics, non-hispanic whites and AA respectively [30]. In spite of the observation that Blacks have mild fibrosis, the rates of HCC and liver cancer-related mortality among Blacks with hepatitis C that has progressed to cirrhosis is higher when compared to Whites [31].

The recognition of these ethnic differences in clinical characteristics, therapeutic response and natural history is important for physicians involved in the care of patients with chronic hepatitis C infection. With the substantial burden of chronic hepatitis C and its sequelae on our healthcare resources, it is imperative that translational studies and clinical trials be designed to better elucidate and understand the underlying pathophysiological mechanisms involved in the observed ethnic differences in this population.

Hepatitis B: Chronic hepatitis B is a leading cause of chronic liver disease and liver-related mortality worldwide. Approximately 350 million people are infected worldwide, with the majority of these occurring in Africa and Asia[32-34]. In the United States, it is estimated that about 1.25 million individuals are chronically infected [35]. Using the NHANES database,

Wasley et al evaluated the prevalence of HBV infection in the era of vaccination. In this study, the age-adjusted prevalence for blacks was 0.89%, non-hispanic-white (0.09%), Mexican Americans (0.07%) and others (0.98%) [36].

To date, eight HBV genotypes (A–H) have been identified worldwide with a prevalence that is dependent on geographic location. Genotype A is the most common form found in the United States and northern Europe, genotypes B and C in Asia, genotype D in the Mediterranean and middle east, genotype E mainly in West Africa, genotype F in Central and South Africa, while the predominant location of genotypes G and H is yet to be clearly determined [37,38]. The clinical significance of the presence of these genotypes in specific geographic locations in relation to ethnicity as well as the influence on the natural history of chronic hepatitis B is not clearly defined. Preliminary studies have revealed that individuals infected with genotypes A and C are associated with a higher prevalence of HBeAg and those with genotype C tend to have a greater likelihood of progression to cirrhosis and HCC with an associated poorer prognosis [38,39]. In regards to treatment, Interferon-based therapies have shown a higher HBeAg seroconversion rate in genotype A- infected individuals, but no consistent association with response rates was found with any of the genotypes in patients treated with nucleoside/nucleotide analogues [40,41]. Further studies are required to elucidate the role of the observed ethnic/geographic variation in genotypes, on treatment response and outcomes [42].

Though the exact prevalence of HBV-HCV coinfection is unknown, a recent study of patients with chronic HCV report a prevalence of 5.8% [43]. Furthermore, they found Asian race to be an independent risk factor for the occurrence of HBV-HCV coinfection. Nguyen et al, also found that among those with HBV-HCV dual infection, the dominant virus in Asians was HBV in contrast to non-Asians in which the HCV was dominant [44]. For HBV-HIV coinfection, results from the HIV outpatient study show a prevalence of 3.5%, 8.7% and 9.5% for Hispanics, Whites and Blacks respectively based on the presence of HBsAg [45]. Important to note that there were no Asians included in the trial thus the prevalence of HBV-HIV coinfection in Asian Americans is unknown. Future studies focusing on the clinical presentation, natural history and therapeutic responses in the coinfected patients (HBV-HCV and HBV-HIV) across ethnic groups will be invaluable.

Non-Alcoholic Fatty Liver Disease: Several recent epidemiologic studies have indicated an increase in the prevalence of NAFLD in the United States. NAFLD is often a hepatic manifestation related to obesity. The marked increase in prevalence within the US is thought to be related to the steady increase in obesity and its associated disorders over the past two decades. Although the rate of obesity has increased across all ethnic groups, there has been a disproportionate increase among black and Hispanic populations. In the United States, the prevalence of NAFLD has been reported to be higher among Hispanics than in other ethnic groups [46-49]. The reason for this difference is unknown but may be related to the higher frequency of the known risk factors for NAFLD among Hispanics. In contrast, the prevalence of NAFLD is lowest in the black population, despite the high rate of risk factors such as diabetes mellitus and obesity within this ethnic group. Recent epidemiologic studies have also found the presence of metabolic syndrome to be a very strong predictor of NAFLD [50]. In the NHANES study, Mexican Americans were found to have the highest prevalence of metabolic syndrome when compared to other ethnic groups [51,52]. This may be contributing, in part, to the higher frequency of NAFLD in individuals of Hispanic ethnicity.

The NAFLD histological spectrum ranges from benign hepatic steatosis to steatohepatitis with or without fibrosis. The natural history and progression of steatohepatitis (i.e., nonalcoholic steatohepatitis) is variable, with diabetes mellitus, obesity, and older age found to be independent predictors of advanced fibrosis and cirrhosis. Several studies have implicated adipokines in the pathogenesis of nonalcoholic steatohepatitis (NASH); in particular, low adiponectin levels have been associated with histologic severity in NASH[53-55]. Ethnic differences in levels of adipokines such as adiponectin and leptin may play a role in the histologic severity of NAFLD [56,57]. The extent to which serum levels of adipokines and/or the presence of metabolic syndrome independently influences disease progression to cirrhosis is uncertain. The current literature suggests that NASH accounts for most cases of cryptogenic cirrhosis but primarily in the Hispanic and Caucasian cohorts [47]. The prevalence of cryptogenic cirrhosis is low in the Black population, and the histologic findings are less severe in this ethnic group than in other ethnic groups [58]. It is unlikely that this difference is due to sampling variability, as these findings of a lower frequency of advanced fibrosis are similar to those observed in blacks with hepatitis C infection. On the contrary, the difference may represent an intrinsic genetic phenomenon in Blacks [59,60]. There is paucity of data on NAFLD in Asian American population. In a small study by Tabibian et al, they report a trend towards severe NASH as measured histologically by steatosis and inflammation in the Asian American group compared to Caucasians [61]. In recent years, there has been a growing interest in the relationship between host related factors and pathogenesis of

NAFLD. The role of host genetic variants such as PNPLA3 and hepatic gene expressions, in NAFLD among different ethnic groups will provide useful insights into the pathogenesis and therapeutic approaches [62-64]. Currently, there are no proven therapies for NAFLD; therefore, the impact of this ethnic variability on therapeutic response is yet to be determined.

Alcohol Liver Disease: Alcoholic liver disease is a common cause of end-stage liver disease in adults. Alcoholic liver disease and its sequelae, ranging from alcoholic hepatitis to Laennec cirrhosis, are well described in the literature. The quantity and type of alcohol consumption that leads to hepatocellular injury are unknown, but studies have identified an association with spirits (distilled alcohol) rather than wine and beer [65,66]. Research has shown that Mexican American and black individuals are more prone to alcohol-induced hepatotoxicity than white individuals [67] Furthermore, Yoon et al analyzed the US Multiple Cause of Death Data and found that mortality rates due to cirrhosis from alcohol and HCV were higher for most Hispanic sub-groups than non-hispanic whites [68]. In addition to this hepatotoxic predisposition, alcohol-cirrhosis related mortality is reported to be higher in Hispanic males than in other ethnic groups [69]. Though the exact reason for this ethnic variation is unknown, it may be related to the type and preference of alcohol consumption as well as the presence of polymorphisms in the different alcohol-metabolizing enzymes [70,71]. Though a recent analysis of the National Vital Statistics shows a significant decline in alcohol liver-related mortality across all ethnic groups over the years, it still represents a significant proportion of liver-related mortality [72]. Therefore, additional studies are needed to further understand the natural history of alcohol liver disease and the role of ethnicity on the predisposition to alcohol-induced hepatotoxicity in the ethnic minority population.

Autoimmune Liver Disease: The most common chronic autoimmune liver disorders are autoimmune hepatitis (AIH), primary sclerosing cholangitis (PSC), and primary biliary cirrhosis (PBC). Of these autoimmune liver disorders, AIH is the most common followed by PBC and PSC. These disorders occur predominantly in white individuals and vary in their progression to end-stage liver disease. There is a paucity of information on the clinical presentation of autoimmune liver disorders in non-white individuals. Case reports of autoimmune hepatitis in non- white individuals suggest that the disease occurs more frequently at an earlier age, with a predominantly cholestatic pattern that is often refractory to standard therapy with prednisone and azathioprine [73-75]. This pattern poses treatment challenges and undoubtedly contributes to disease progression. The exact mechanism underlying this distinct clinical presentation and outcome has yet to be determined. The interrelationship between ethnicity, genetics, and individual HLA phenotype may provide useful insight into this observation. Though prevalence and clinical characteristics of the cholestatic diseases (PSC and PBC) in non-white individuals has not been fully investigated, Peters et al found that non-Caucasians (Hispanic and AA) with PBC presented with more severe disease than Caucasians [76]. Future clinical studies involving enrollment of participants of diverse ethnicity will provide an insight into the understanding of the complex inter-relationship between ethnicity, autoimmunity and the environment.

Hepatocellular Carcinoma: Hepatocellular carcinoma is the most common primary liver cancer worldwide. The prevalence of HCC the United States continues to increase, particularly in the black population, for which the incidence is two-fold higher than that of the white population [77]. Clinical presentation and tumor stage at the time of diagnosis also appears to be influenced by ethnicity, with black patients and Latinos having more advanced tumors at the time of diagnosis [78,79]. Ethnicity also has been shown to impact the diagnostic utility of non-invasive tumor markers, such as alpha-fetoprotein (AFP). Serum AFP has been found to have a low sensitivity as a tumor marker among black patients with cirrhosis, thereby diminishing its clinical utility in this population [80]. However, the impact of ethnicity on the predictive value of other diagnostic markers such as AFP-L3 and des-gamma-carboxyprothrombin (DCP) is unknown. In addition to the observed ethnic differences on the clinical profile of HCC, the role of ethnicity on the available therapeutic approaches has been reported. Access and utilization of surgical and non-surgical therapies for HCC varies by race/ethnicity, with a lower likelihood reported for ethnic minorities [81-83]. Furthermore, significant ethnic variations in survival have been reported, with lower overall survival for Blacks and Hispanics compared to Whites [4,84]. In order to fully understand the interaction between ethnicity and HCC, the impact of socioeconomic status and access to health care on the observed racial disparities needs to be investigated further.

Conclusion

Due to our ethnically diverse population and the disproportionate rate of chronic liver diseases amongst minorities, a better understanding of the impact of ethnicity/race is essential in order to identify strategies that will decrease prevalence of preventable liver diseases and ultimately improve therapeutic outcomes in this population. Though this review summarizes the complex relationship between ethnicity and liver disease, it also highlights the lack of population-based studies with adequate representation of all ethnic groups. The significance of adequate representation of currently underrepresented ethnic minorities in clinical trials and the consistent reporting and classification of race/ethnicity in population-based studies cannot be overemphasized. In conclusion, ethnic differences exist in chronic liver disease and in some instances influences treatment outcomes and overall prognosis. A heightened awareness of these ethnic variations is important for the practicing healthcare provider. Future research strategies into the increased morbidity and mortality amongst the various minority ethnic groups will help clarify and improve the ethnic differences in chronic liver disease.

References

[1] Khokhar OS, Lewis JH: Reasons why patients infected with chronic hepatitis c virus choose to defer treatment: Do they alter their decision with time? D*ig. Dis. Sci*. 2007;52:1168-1176.

[2] Trooskin SB, Navarro VJ, Winn RJ, Axelrod DJ, McNeal AS, Velez M, Herrine SK, Rossi S: Hepatitis c risk assessment, testing and referral for treatment in urban primary care: Role of race and ethnicity. *World J. Gastroenterol* 2007;13:1074-1078.

[3] Nguyen GC, Segev DL, Thuluvath PJ: Racial disparities in the management of hospitalized patients with cirrhosis and complications of portal hypertension: A national study. *Hepatology* 2007;45:1282-1289.

[4] Davila JA, El-Serag HB: Racial differences in survival of hepatocellular carcinoma in the united states: A population-based study. *Clin. Gastroenterol. Hepatol*. 2006;4:104-110; quiz 104-105.

[5] Armstrong GL, Wasley A, Simard EP, McQuillan GM, Kuhnert WL, Alter MJ: The prevalence of hepatitis c virus infection in the united states, 1999 through 2002. *Ann. Intern Med*. 2006;144:705-714.

[6] Nainan OV, Alter MJ, Kruszon-Moran D, Gao FX, Xia G, McQuillan G, Margolis HS: Hepatitis c virus genotypes and viral concentrations in participants of a general population survey in the united states. *Gastroenterology* 2006;131:478-484.

[7] Conjeevaram HS, Fried MW, Jeffers LJ, Terrault NA, Wiley-Lucas TE, Afdhal N, Brown RS, Belle SH, Hoofnagle JH, Kleiner DE, Howell CD: Peginterferon and ribavirin treatment in african american and caucasian american patients with hepatitis c genotype 1. *Gastroenterology* 2006;131:470-477.

[8] Muir AJ, Bornstein JD, Killenberg PG: Peginterferon alfa-2b and ribavirin for the treatment of chronic hepatitis c in blacks and non-hispanic whites. *N. Engl. J. Med.* 2004;350:2265-2271.

[9] Rodriguez-Torres M, Jeffers LJ, Sheikh MY, Rossaro L, Ankoma-Sey V, Hamzeh FM, Martin P: Peginterferon alfa-2a and ribavirin in latino and non-latino whites with hepatitis c. *N. Engl. J. Med.* 2009;360:257-267.

[10] Muir AJ, Hu KQ, Gordon SC, Koury K, Boparai N, Noviello S, Albrecht JK, Sulkowski MS, McCone J: Hepatitis c treatment among racial and ethnic groups in the ideal trial. *J. Viral. Hepat*;18:e134-143.

[11] Shiffman ML, Mihas AA, Millwala F, Sterling RK, Luketic VA, Stravitz RT, Sanyal AJ: Treatment of chronic hepatitis c virus in african americans with genotypes 2 and 3. *Am. J. Gastroenterol* 2007;102:761-766.

[12] Poordad F, McCone J, Jr., Bacon BR, Bruno S, Manns MP, Sulkowski MS, Jacobson IM, Reddy KR, Goodman ZD, Boparai N, DiNubile MJ, Sniukiene V, Brass CA, Albrecht JK, Bronowicki JP: Boceprevir for untreated chronic hcv genotype 1 infection. *N. Engl. J. Med.*;364:1195-1206.

[13] Jacobson IM, McHutchison JG, Dusheiko G, Di Bisceglie AM, Reddy KR, Bzowej NH, Marcellin P, Muir AJ, Ferenci P, Flisiak R, George J, Rizzetto M, Shouval D, Sola R, Terg RA, Yoshida EM, Adda N, Bengtsson L, Sankoh AJ, Kieffer TL, George S, Kauffman RS, Zeuzem S: Telaprevir for previously untreated chronic hepatitis c virus infection. *N. Engl. J. Med.*;364:2405-2416.

[14] Zeuzem S, Andreone P, Pol S, Lawitz E, Diago M, Roberts S, Focaccia R, Younossi Z, Foster GR, Horban A, Ferenci P, Nevens F, Mullhaupt B, Pockros P, Terg R, Shouval D, van Hoek B, Weiland O, Van Heeswijk R, De Meyer S, Luo D, Boogaerts G, Polo R, Picchio G, Beumont M: Telaprevir for retreatment of hcv infection. *N. Engl. J. Med.*;364:2417-2428.

[15] Bacon BR, Gordon SC, Lawitz E, Marcellin P, Vierling JM, Zeuzem S, Poordad F, Goodman ZD, Sings HL, Boparai N, Burroughs M, Brass

CA, Albrecht JK, Esteban R: Boceprevir for previously treated chronic hcv genotype 1 infection. *N. Engl. J. Med.*;364:1207-1217.

[16] Kimball P, Elswick RK, Shiffman M: Ethnicity and cytokine production gauge response of patients with hepatitis c to interferon-alpha therapy. *J. Med. Virol.* 2001;65:510-516.

[17] Sugimoto K, Stadanlick J, Ikeda F, Brensinger C, Furth EE, Alter HJ, Chang KM: Influence of ethnicity in the outcome of hepatitis c virus infection and cellular immune response. *Hepatology* 2003;37:590-599.

[18] Ge D, Fellay J, Thompson AJ, Simon JS, Shianna KV, Urban TJ, Heinzen EL, Qiu P, Bertelsen AH, Muir AJ, Sulkowski M, McHutchison JG, Goldstein DB: Genetic variation in il28b predicts hepatitis c treatment-induced viral clearance. *Nature* 2009;461:399-401.

[19] Thomas DL, Thio CL, Martin MP, Qi Y, Ge D, O'Huigin C, Kidd J, Kidd K, Khakoo SI, Alexander G, Goedert JJ, Kirk GD, Donfield SM, Rosen HR, Tobler LH, Busch MP, McHutchison JG, Goldstein DB, Carrington M: Genetic variation in il28b and spontaneous clearance of hepatitis c virus. *Nature* 2009;461:798-801.

[20] Conjeevaram HS, Kleiner DE, Everhart JE, Hoofnagle JH, Zacks S, Afdhal NH, Wahed AS: Race, insulin resistance and hepatic steatosis in chronic hepatitis c. *Hepatology* 2007;45:80-87.

[21] Cheung RC, Currie S, Shen H, Ho SB, Bini EJ, Anand BS, Brau N, Wright TL: Chronic hepatitis c in latinos: Natural history, treatment eligibility, acceptance, and outcomes. *Am. J. Gastroenterol.* 2005;100:2186-2193.

[22] Harrison SA, Brunt EM, Qazi RA, Oliver DA, Neuschwander-Tetri BA, Di Bisceglie AM, Bacon BR: Effect of significant histologic steatosis or steatohepatitis on response to antiviral therapy in patients with chronic hepatitis c. *Clin. Gastroenterol. Hepatol.* 2005;3:604-609.

[23] Hu KQ, Currie SL, Shen H, Cheung RC, Ho SB, Bini EJ, McCracken JD, Morgan T, Brau N, Schmidt WN, Jeffers L, Wright TL: Clinical implications of hepatic steatosis in patients with chronic hepatitis c: A multicenter study of u.S. Veterans. *Dig. Dis. Sci.* 2007;52:570-578.

[24] Soresi M, Tripi S, Franco V, Giannitrapani L, Alessandri A, Rappa F, Vuturo O, Montalto G: Impact of liver steatosis on the antiviral response in the hepatitis c virus-associated chronic hepatitis. *Liver Int* 2006;26:1119-1125.

[25] Sterling RK, Salvatori JJ, Luketic VA, Sanyal AJ, Fulcher AS, Stravitz RT, Contos MJ, Mills AS, Shiffman ML: A prospective, randomized-controlled pilot study of ursodeoxycholic acid combined with

mycophenolate mofetil in the treatment of primary sclerosing cholangitis. *Aliment. Pharmacol. Ther*. 2004;20:943-949.

[26] Crosse K, Umeadi OG, Anania FA, Laurin J, Papadimitriou J, Drachenberg C, Howell CD: Racial differences in liver inflammation and fibrosis related to chronic hepatitis c. *Clin. Gastroenterol. Hepatol.* 2004;2:463-468.

[27] Lepe R, Layden-Almer JE, Layden TJ, Cotler S: Ethnic differences in the presentation of chronic hepatitis c. *J. Viral. Hepat*. 2006;13:116-120.

[28] Verma S, Bonacini M, Govindarajan S, Kanel G, Lindsay KL, Redeker A: More advanced hepatic fibrosis in hispanics with chronic hepatitis c infection: Role of patient demographics, hepatic necroinflammation, and steatosis. *Am. J. Gastroenterol*. 2006;101:1817-1823.

[29] Wiley TE, Brown J, Chan J: Hepatitis c infection in african americans: Its natural history and histological progression. *Am. J. Gastroenterol.* 2002;97:700-706.

[30] Kallwitz ER, Layden-Almer J, Dhamija M, Berkes J, Guzman G, Lepe R, Cotler SJ, Layden TJ: Ethnicity and body mass index are associated with hepatitis c presentation and progression. *Clin. Gastroenterol. Hepatol.*;8:72-78.

[31] Pearlman BL: Hepatitis c virus infection in african americans. *Clin. Infect Dis*. 2006;42:82-91.

[32] Lavanchy D: Hepatitis b virus epidemiology, disease burden, treatment, and current and emerging prevention and control measures. *J. Viral. Hepat.* 2004;11:97-107.

[33] McQuillan GM, Coleman PJ, Kruszon-Moran D, Moyer LA, Lambert SB, Margolis HS: Prevalence of hepatitis b virus infection in the united states: The national health and nutrition examination surveys, 1976 through 1994. *Am. J. Public Health* 1999;89:14-18.

[34] Kramvis A, Kew MC: Epidemiology of hepatitis b virus in africa, its genotypes and clinical associations of genotypes. *Hepatol. Res.* 2007;37:S9-S19.

[35] Gish RG, Gadano AC: Chronic hepatitis b: Current epidemiology in the americas and implications for management. *J. Viral Hepat.* 2006;13:787-798.

[36] Wasley A, Kruszon-Moran D, Kuhnert W, Simard EP, Finelli L, McQuillan G, Bell B: The prevalence of hepatitis b virus infection in the united states in the era of vaccination. *J. Infect. Dis*;202:192-201.

[37] Liu CJ, Kao JH, Chen DS: Therapeutic implications of hepatitis b virus genotypes. *Liver Int.* 2005;25:1097-1107.

[38] Chu CJ, Keeffe EB, Han SH, Perrillo RP, Min AD, Soldevila-Pico C, Carey W, Brown RS, Jr., Luketic VA, Terrault N, Lok AS: Hepatitis b virus genotypes in the united states: Results of a nationwide study. *Gastroenterology* 2003;125:444-451.

[39] Kao JH, Chen PJ, Lai MY, Chen DS: Hepatitis b genotypes correlate with clinical outcomes in patients with chronic hepatitis b. *Gastroenterology* 2000;118:554-559.

[40] Kao JH, Wu NH, Chen PJ, Lai MY, Chen DS: Hepatitis b genotypes and the response to interferon therapy. *J. Hepatol.* 2000;33:998-1002.

[41] Janssen HL, van Zonneveld M, Senturk H, Zeuzem S, Akarca US, Cakaloglu Y, Simon C, So TM, Gerken G, de Man RA, Niesters HG, Zondervan P, Hansen B, Schalm SW: Pegylated interferon alfa-2b alone or in combination with lamivudine for hbeag-positive chronic hepatitis b: A randomised trial. *Lancet* 2005;365:123-129.

[42] Chu CJ, Keeffe EB, Han SH, Perrillo RP, Min AD, Soldevila-Pico C, Carey W, Brown RS, Jr., Luketic VA, Terrault N, Lok AS: Prevalence of hbv precore/core promoter variants in the united states. *Hepatology* 2003;38:619-628.

[43] Bini EJ, Perumalswami PV: Hepatitis b virus infection among american patients with chronic hepatitis c virus infection: Prevalence, racial/ethnic differences, and viral interactions. *Hepatology*;51:759-766.

[44] Nguyen LH, Ko S, Wong SS, Tran PS, Trinh HN, Garcia RT, Ahmed A, Lutchman GA, Keeffe EB, Nguyen MH: Ethnic differences in viral dominance patterns in patients with hepatitis b virus and hepatitis c virus dual infection. *Hepatology;*53:1839-1845.

[45] Spradling PR, Richardson JT, Buchacz K, Moorman AC, Brooks JT: Prevalence of chronic hepatitis b virus infection among patients in the hiv outpatient study, 1996-2007. *J. Viral Hepat.*

[46] Weston SR, Leyden W, Murphy R, Bass NM, Bell BP, Manos MM, Terrault NA: Racial and ethnic distribution of nonalcoholic fatty liver in persons with newly diagnosed chronic liver disease. *Hepatology* 2005;41:372-379.

[47] Browning JD, Kumar KS, Saboorian MH, Thiele DL: Ethnic differences in the prevalence of cryptogenic cirrhosis. *Am. J. Gastroenterol.* 2004;99:292-298.

[48] Browning JD, Szczepaniak LS, Dobbins R, Nuremberg P, Horton JD, Cohen JC, Grundy SM, Hobbs HH: Prevalence of hepatic steatosis in an urban population in the united states: Impact of ethnicity. *Hepatology* 2004;40:1387-1395.

[49] Caldwell SH, Harris DM, Patrie JT, Hespenheide EE: Is nash underdiagnosed among african americans? *Am. J. Gastroenterol.* 2002;97:1496-1500.

[50] Hamaguchi M, Kojima T, Takeda N, Nakagawa T, Taniguchi H, Fujii K, Omatsu T, Nakajima T, Sarui H, Shimazaki M, Kato T, Okuda J, Ida K: The metabolic syndrome as a predictor of nonalcoholic fatty liver disease. *Ann. Intern. Med.* 2005;143:722-728.

[51] Ford ES, Giles WH, Dietz WH: Prevalence of the metabolic syndrome among us adults: Findings from the third national health and nutrition examination survey. *JAMA* 2002;287:356-359.

[52] Park YW, Zhu S, Palaniappan L, Heshka S, Carnethon MR, Heymsfield SB: The metabolic syndrome: Prevalence and associated risk factor findings in the us population from the third national health and nutrition examination survey, 1988-1994. *Arch. Intern. Med.* 2003;163:427-436.

[53] Musso G, Gambino R, Biroli G, Carello M, Faga E, Pacini G, De Michieli F, Cassader M, Durazzo M, Rizzetto M, Pagano G: Hypoadiponectinemia predicts the severity of hepatic fibrosis and pancreatic beta-cell dysfunction in nondiabetic nonobese patients with nonalcoholic steatohepatitis. *Am. J. Gastroenterol.* 2005;100:2438-2446.

[54] Vuppalanchi R, Marri S, Kolwankar D, Considine RV, Chalasani N: Is adiponectin involved in the pathogenesis of nonalcoholic steatohepatitis? A preliminary human study. *J. Clin. Gastroenterol.* 2005;39:237-242.

[55] Kaser S, Moschen A, Cayon A, Kaser A, Crespo J, Pons-Romero F, Ebenbichler CF, Patsch JR, Tilg H: Adiponectin and its receptors in non-alcoholic steatohepatitis. *Gut* 2005;54:117-121.

[56] Hulver MW, Saleh O, MacDonald KG, Pories WJ, Barakat HA: Ethnic differences in adiponectin levels. *Metabolism* 2004;53:1-3.

[57] Ruhl CE, Everhart JE: Leptin concentrations in the united states: Relations with demographic and anthropometric measures. *Am. J. Clin. Nutr.* 2001;74:295-301.

[58] Solga SF, Clark JM, Alkhuraishi AR, Torbenson M, Tabesh A, Schweitzer M, Diehl AM, Magnuson TH: Race and comorbid factors predict nonalcoholic fatty liver disease histopathology in severely obese patients. *Surg. Obes. Relat Dis.* 2005;1:6-11.

[59] Ratziu V, Poynard T: Assessing the outcome of nonalcoholic steatohepatitis? It's time to get serious. *Hepatology* 2006;44:802-805.

[60] Merriman RB, Ferrell LD, Patti MG, Weston SR, Pabst MS, Aouizerat BE, Bass NM: Correlation of paired liver biopsies in morbidly obese

patients with suspected nonalcoholic fatty liver disease. *Hepatology* 2006;44:874-880.

[61] Tabibian JH, Lazo M, Durazo FA, Yeh HC, Tong MJ, Clark JM: Nonalcoholic fatty liver disease across ethno-racial groups: Do asian-american adults represent a new at-risk population? *J. Gastroenterol. Hepatol;*26:501-509.

[62] Wagenknecht LE, Palmer ND, Bowden DW, Rotter JI, Norris JM, Ziegler J, Chen YD, Haffner S, Scherzinger A, Langefeld CD: Association of pnpla3 with non-alcoholic fatty liver disease in a minority cohort: The insulin resistance atherosclerosis family study. *Liver Int*;31:412-416.

[63] Stepanova M, Hossain N, Afendy A, Perry K, Goodman ZD, Baranova A, Younossi Z: Hepatic gene expression of caucasian and african-american patients with obesity-related non-alcoholic fatty liver disease. *Obes. Surg.;*20:640-650.

[64] Romeo S, Kozlitina J, Xing C, Pertsemlidis A, Cox D, Pennacchio LA, Boerwinkle E, Cohen JC, Hobbs HH: Genetic variation in pnpla3 confers susceptibility to nonalcoholic fatty liver disease. *Nat. Genet* 2008;40:1461-1465.

[65] Becker U, Deis A, Sorensen TI, Gronbaek M, Borch-Johnsen K, Muller CF, Schnohr P, Jensen G: Prediction of risk of liver disease by alcohol intake, sex, and age: A prospective population study. *Hepatology* 1996;23:1025-1029.

[66] Gronbaek M, Becker U, Johansen D, Gottschau A, Schnohr P, Hein HO, Jensen G, Sorensen TI: Type of alcohol consumed and mortality from all causes, coronary heart disease, and cancer. *Ann. Intern. Med.* 2000;133:411-419.

[67] Stewart SH: Racial and ethnic differences in alcohol-associated aspartate aminotransferase and gamma-glutamyltransferase elevation. *Arch. Intern. Med.* 2002;162:2236-2239.

[68] Yoon YH, Yi HY, Thomson PC: Alcohol-related and viral hepatitis c-related cirrhosis mortality among hispanic subgroups in the united states, 2000-2004. *Alcohol. Clin. Exp. Res.*;35:240-249.

[69] Stinson FS, Grant BF, Dufour MC: The critical dimension of ethnicity in liver cirrhosis mortality statistics. *Alcohol. Clin. Exp. Res.* 2001;25:1181-1187.

[70] Zintzaras E, Stefanidis I, Santos M, Vidal F: Do alcohol-metabolizing enzyme gene polymorphisms increase the risk of alcoholism and alcoholic liver disease? *Hepatology* 2006;43:352-361.

[71] Lorenzo A, Auguet T, Vidal F, Broch M, Olona M, Gutierrez C, Lopez-Dupla M, Sirvent JJ, Quer JC, Santos M, Richart C: Polymorphisms of alcohol-metabolizing enzymes and the risk for alcoholism and alcoholic liver disease in caucasian spanish women. *Drug Alcohol. Depend* 2006;84:195-200.

[72] Paula H, Asrani SK, Boetticher NC, Pedersen R, Shah VH, Kim WR: Alcoholic liver disease-related mortality in the united states: 1980-2003. *Am. J. Gastroenterol*;105:1782-1787.

[73] Zolfino T, Heneghan MA, Norris S, Harrison PM, Portmann BC, McFarlane IG: Characteristics of autoimmune hepatitis in patients who are not of european caucasoid ethnic origin. *Gut* 2002;50:713-717.

[74] Lim KN, Casanova RL, Boyer TD, Bruno CJ: Autoimmune hepatitis in african americans: Presenting features and response to therapy. *Am. J. Gastroenterol.* 2001;96:3390-3394.

[75] D'Souza R, Sinnott P, Glynn MJ, Sabin CA, Foster GR: An unusual form of autoimmune hepatitis in young somalian men. *Liver Int* 2005;25:325-330.

[76] Peters MG, Di Bisceglie AM, Kowdley KV, Flye NL, Luketic VA, Munoz SJ, Garcia-Tsao G, Boyer TD, Lake JR, Bonacini M, Combes B: Differences between caucasian, african american, and hispanic patients with primary biliary cirrhosis in the united states. *Hepatology* 2007;46:769-775.

[77] McGlynn KA, Tarone RE, El-Serag HB: A comparison of trends in the incidence of hepatocellular carcinoma and intrahepatic cholangiocarcinoma in the united states. *Cancer Epidemiol Biomarkers Prev.* 2006;15:1198-1203.

[78] Guerrero-Preston R, Siegel A, Renz J, Vlahov D, Neugut A: Hcv infection and cryptogenic cirrhosis are risk factors for hepatocellular carcinoma among latinos in new york city. *J. Community Health* 2009;34:500-505.

[79] Kemmer N, Neff G, Secic M, Zacharias V, Kaiser T, Buell J: Ethnic differences in hepatocellular carcinoma: Implications for liver transplantation. *Dig. Dis Sci.* 2008;53:551-555.

[80] Nguyen MH, Garcia RT, Simpson PW, Wright TL, Keeffe EB: Racial differences in effectiveness of alpha-fetoprotein for diagnosis of hepatocellular carcinoma in hepatitis c virus cirrhosis. *Hepatology* 2002;36:410-417.

[81] Robbins AS, Daily MF, Aoki CA, Chen MS, Jr., Troppmann C, Perez RV: Decreasing disparity in liver transplantation among white and asian

patients with hepatocellular carcinoma : California, 1998-2005. *Cancer* 2008;113:2173-2179.

[82] Zak Y, Rhoads KF, Visser BC: Predictors of surgical intervention for hepatocellular carcinoma: Race, socioeconomic status, and hospital type. *Arch. Surg;*146:778-784.

[83] Siegel AB, McBride RB, El-Serag HB, Hershman DL, Brown RS, Jr., Renz JF, Emond J, Neugut AI: Racial disparities in utilization of liver transplantation for hepatocellular carcinoma in the united states, 1998-2002. *Am. J. Gastroenterol.* 2008;103:120-127.

[84] Harrison LE, Reichman T, Koneru B, Fisher A, Wilson D, Dela Torre A, Samanta A, Korogodsky M: Racial discrepancies in the outcome of patients with hepatocellular carcinoma. *Arch. Surg.* 2004;139:992-996.

In: Liver Disease and Peritonitis
Editor: Mao Kang Voung et al.
ISBN 978-1-61942-080-9

Chapter 5

Alteration of Adhesion Molecules Expression and Cellular Polarity in Liver Diseases

*Yi Cao**, *Hong Chang and Chen Zhang*
Laboratory of Molecular and Experimental Pathology,
Key Laboratory of Animal Models and Human Disease Mechanism of CAS and Yunnan Province, Kunming Institute of Zoology,
Chinese Academy of Sciences, Peoples' Republic of China

Abstract

The expression of the adhesion molecules in normal liver tissues, benign including probable premalignant lesions, and malignant lesions was systematically investigated in our previous study. In a normal liver, both hepatocytes and bile duct cells expressedtight junction proteins (ZO-1, symplekin), adherens junction proteins (E-cadherin, α-catenin, β-catenin, γ-catenin), and desmosome proteins (desmoglein 1/2, desmocollin 2, desmoplakin, and plakophilin 2), but did not express some

*Address for correspondence: Prof. Dr. Yi Cao, Laboratory of Molecular and Experimental Pathology, Kunming Institute of Zoology, Chinese Academy of Sciences, 32 Jiaochang Donglu, Kunming, Yunnan 650223, Peoples' Republic of China, Tel.: 0086-871-5199081, Fax: 0086-871-5199081, E-mail: caoy@mail.kiz.ac.cn

desmosome proteinssuch as desmocollin 1/3 and plakophilin 1. In the benign hepatocyte lesions, expression of the adherens junctions and the desmosomes was uniform and slightly increased, but symplekin appeared in a reduced expression in dysplastic lesions. In hepatocellular carcinomas (HCCs), expression of the adhesion molecules was often heterogeneous and in an abnormal location. Tumor cells with an abnormal distribution or loss of adhesion molecules show an apolar arrangement oftissue architecture. The expression levels of the adhesion molecules correlated with the differentiation grades of HCC. Furthermore, we found that abnormal expression of symplekin was involved in the loss of cellular polarity, the increased permeability of epithelial monolayers, and the change of cellular proliferation in vitro. Alteration of adhesion molecules and cellular polarity plays pathophysiological roles in the development and progress of hepatocellular carcinomas: (1) Abnormal location and decrease/loss of the adhesion molecules in cancer cells may reduce the adherence of hepatocytes to their neighboring cells. These functions might cause or promote invasive growth of tumor cells; (2) Some adhesion molecules (e.g. ZO-1 and β-catenin) are associated with signal transduction. Abnormal expression and distribution of the adhesion molecules may interfere with normal signal transduction and cell proliferation;(3) Adhesion molecules of epithelial cells play an important role in maintaining cellular polarity. Because of loss of polarity in cancer cells due to reduction of the adherence between hepatocytes, other adhesion molecules e.g. integrins and CD44, could be located anywhere on the cell surface of apolar cancer cells instead of its restricted domain localization in normal cells and might allow aberrant binding to the extracellular matrix and endothelial cells.

In addition, some adhesion moleculessuch as E-cadherin, desmoglein 1, desmoglein 2, desmocollin 2, desmoplakin, and plakophilin 2, are tightly restricted to the epithelial constituents in a normal liver and in various liver diseases, but are completely lacking in hematopoietic and endothelial cells. These epithelial cell-specific adhesion molecules could be applied as targets to detect carcinoma cells in blood or bone marrow for early detection of HCC and for prognosis of metastases.

Keywords: tight junction, adherens junctions, desmosomes, liver, tumor

Hepatocellular carcinomas (HCCs) are one of the major human cancers. The concept of tumorigenesis as a multistep process is widely accepted. The accumulation of genetic changes is assumed to be responsible for successive waves of clonal expansion of transformed cells. Models of tumor progression provide an excellent opportunity to study genetic, cellular, biochemical, and immunological alterations that occur during this process and to assess their importance and possible functional role during malignant transformation. A model of hepatocarcinogenesis has not yet been completely established. However, possible precursor lesions of HCC have been increasingly recognized in the past one or two decades [International Working Party, 1995]. Hepatocellular dysplastic lesions caused by presumed genetic alteration represent probable premalignant changes. It is of interest to compare the expression of biologically active adhesion molecules in normal hepatocytes, benign including probable premalignant lesions, and malignantlesions in order to study their roles during hepatocarcinogenesis.

Cell adhesion is of fundamental importance in normal morphogenesis and neoplastic transformation of epithelial cells [Lecuit, 2005]. Adhesion molecules of epithelial cells include tight junctions, adherens junctions, and desmosomes. Tight junctionsin polarized epithelia form regular intercellular barriers between epithelial cells. They prevent paracellular transport of molecules and particles and separate distinct apical and basolateral plasma membrane surfaces. Adherens junctions are complex structures and contain the transmembrane glycoprotein E-cadherin and three submembranous cytosolic proteins, α-catenin, β-catenin, and γ-catenin. E-cadherin molecules form lateral, parallel dimers on the cell surface. The parallel dimers interdigitate with dimers from adjacent cells to form the point of adhesion. On the cytoplasmic side of the membrane, E-cadherin interacts with either β-catenin or γ-catenin, and α-catenin links the bound β- or γ-catenin to the actin cytoskeleton [Birchmeier, 1995]. Desmosomes are punctate membrane domains traversed by representatives of two types of desmosomal cadherins, desmogleins and desmoncollins, whose cytoplasmic tails contribute to a dense plaque containing plakoglobin (γ-catenin), desmoplakin, and plakophilin that anchor the intermediate filaments [Garrod et al, 1996; Mertens et al, 1996]. Unlike the adherens junctions and desmosomes, the tight junction has a very complicated protein composition. Over the past three decays, a number of proteins have been found to localize to the tight junction complex, including claudin 1-24, occludin, tricellulin, junctional adhesion molecule (JAM), ZO-1-3, ZO-1-associated nucleic acid binding protein (ZONAB), cingulin, and symplekin [Franke, 2009]. The claudin family membrane proteins interact with each other between cells to generate the tight junction strands. Occludin, tricellulin, and JAM are also localized at the tight junction strands. ZO-1-3, ZONAB, cingulin, and symplekin are localized on the cytoplasmic side of the tight junction strands. ZO family proteins bind to the C-terminal cytoplasmic domain of claudins, occluding, tricellulin, and JAM. ZO-1-3 and cingulin interact with F-actin. [Furuse, 2010]. Adhesion molecules of epithelial cells contributed to cell-cell attachment and coherence, and are involved in signal transduction and maintaining cellular polarity. Alterations of adhesion molecules have be shown to contribute not only to the later stages of tumor progression such as invasion and metastatic spread, but also to early functional changes that transform a normal epithelial cell into a carcinoma cell [Perl et al, 1998]. Here we provided a systematic and comprehensive overview on the expression of adhesion molecules in a normal human liver and in various liver diseases, including cirrhosis, metabolic diseases, and hepatocellular neoplasia.

Polarity is a very important character of epithelial cells. Many factors are involved inthe polarity, such as adhesion molecules, cytoskeletal arrangement, membrane domains-specific intracellular transport, and so on. Loss of polarity is an important feature of malignant transformation [Cao et al, 1997]. The hepatocyte is a polarized epithelial cell whose surface is composed of three functionally and morphologically distinct domains—the sinusoidal membrane, the lateral membrane, and the bile canalicular membrane (the apical membrane) [Hubbard et al, 1983]. The sinusoidal membrane is specialized for exchange of metabolites with the blood. The lateral membrane, which is contiguous to a neighboring hepatocyte, is adapted for cell attachment and cell-cell communication, and thus is marked by junctional elements. The bile canalicular membrane, which is separated from the lateral membrane by tight junctions, is specialized for bile secretion. An apolar arrangement has been regarded as a key step in the process of hepatocarcinogenesis [Stamatoglou et al, 1994]. Adhesion molecules of epithelial cells play an important role in keeping cellular polarity. In the chapter, alteration of cellular polarity in HCCs has also been discussed.

1. Expression of Adhesion Molecules in the Normal Liver

In normal liver tissues, both hepatocytes and bile duct cells showed homogeneous expression of symplekin, E-cadherin, α-catenin, β-catenin, γ-catenin, desmoglein 1, desmoglein 2, desmocollin 2, desmoplakin, and plakophilin 2. Desmocollin 1, desmocollin 3, and plakophilin 1 were not expressed in the liver. The tight junction proteins, ZO-1 and symplekin, were expressed along the apical membrane of biliary epithelial cells and along the bile canaliculi of hepatocytes [Ihara et al, 1996; Cao et al, 2007].

Others cell and tissue types, such as Kupffer cells, fat-storing cells, sinusoidal endothelial cells, vascular endothelial cells, lymphocytes, nerve, connective tissue, and vascular muscles did not express E-cadherin, desmoglein 1, desmoglein 2, desmocollin 1, desmocollin 2, desmoplakin, plakophilin 1, and plakophilin 2. Immunopositivity for α-catenin, β-catenin, and γ-catenin was also found in vascular endothelial cells and nerve bundles in the portal tracts, but not in Kupffer cells, fat-storing cells, sinusoidal endothelial cells, lymphocytes, connective tissue, and vascular muscles [Cao et al, 2007].

2. Expression of Adhesion Molecules in Cirrhotic Liver and Liver Cell Adenomas

In the regenerative lesions of the liver cirrhosis, expression of adherens junctions (E-cadherin, α-catenin, β-catenin, and γ-catenin) and desmosomes (desmoglein 1 and 2, desmocollin 2, desmoplakin, and plakophilin 2) was uniform and slightly increased as compared with that of the normal hepatocytes. The distribution of these adhesion molecules was unchanged. The proliferated oval cells and the pseudotubules strongly expressed the tight junction (symplekin), the adherens junctions, the desmosomes. In hepatic glycogenoses, the patterns of immunoreactivity of the adhesion molecules were similar to those observed in the normal liver [Cao et al, 2007].

The dysplastic lesions were considered putatively premalignant lesions frequently associated with cirrhosis and HCC [International Working Party, 1995]. The expression of the adherens junctions (E-cadherin, α-catenin, β-catenin, and γ-catenin) and the desmosomes (desmoglein 1 and 2, desmocollin 2, desmoplakin, and plakophilin 2) in the dysplastic hepatocytes and the adenomas was similar to that observed in the regenerative lesions. However, the expression of symplekin in the dysplastic lesions was no longer uniform and some bile canaliculi showed no presence of the tight junction [Cao et al, 2007].

3. Expression of Adhesion Molecules in HCCs

Changes in the expression of E-cadherin, α-catenin, β-catenin, and γ-catenin have been observed in the neoplasm of various tissues [Inagawa et al, 2002; Kozyraki et al, 1996; Ihara et al, 1996]. In previous studies, we investigated systematically the expression of tight junction (symplekin), adherens junctions (E-cadherin, α-catenin, β-catenin, γ-catenin), and desmosomes (desmoglein 1, 2; desmocollin 1, 2, 3; desmoplakin; plakophilin 1, 2) in malignant lesions of hepatocytes [Cao et al, 2007]. Instead of the regular expression of the adherens junctions and the desmosomes in normal hepatocytes and benign hepatocellular lesions, HCCs displayed irregular distribution of these adhesion molecules at the total plasma membrane and/or in the diffuse cytoplasm of tumor cells. Nuclear staining for β-catenin was also observed in some cases. The expression levels of the adherens junctions and desmosomes in different samples were polymorphous. Within a given tumor, the cancer cells showed heterogeneous expression, ranging from none to very high amounts per cell, different from normal hepatocytes present in the adjacent peritumoral tissue. These alterations may be explained by tumor cell polymorphism with simultaneous up-regulation and down-regulation of the adhesion molecules, as well as abnormal intracellular transport and distribution of the proteins. We also found the abnormal expression of these adhesion molecules in human gastrointestinal carcinomas similar to HCCs [Zhang et al, 2011].

The expression levels of the adherens junctions and the desmosomes correlated with the grades of differentiation of HCC cells. In well and moderately differentiated HCCs, a part of the tumor cells showed markedly lower expression of the adherens junctions and the desmosomes. In contrast, most or even almost all cancer cells lost the ability to express the adherens junctions and the desmosomes in poorly differentiated HCCs.

The adherens junction molecules (E-cadherin, α-catenin, β-catenin, and γ-catenin) and the desmosome molecules (desmoglein 1 and 2, desmocollin 2, desmoplakin, and plakophilin 2) are closely related molecules, these molecules together assemble the functional complexes — the adherens junction and desmosome, respectively. The simultaneous expression of the adherens junctions and the desmosomes in the same cell was examined in our previous study. We observed a correlation between the adherens junction molecules with respect to the intensity of reactivity in most tumor cells (tumor cells strongly positive for one molecule were also intensely immunoreactive for others and vice versa). However, it was also noted in our serial immunohistochemical preparations that in several cases, especially in poorly differentiated HCCs, some cancer cells showed the complementary expression of the adherens junction molecules (e.g. there were cells expressing E-cadherin and lacking the catenins, but the latter could be found on another subset of cells). Similarly, both phenomena — the close relationship in the majority of tumor cells and the discrepant expression in the minority of tumor cells — were also observed in the expression of the desmosomes. This indicated that these molecules are not able to assemble the functional complexes in the cancer cells despite their existence. Normal desmosome assembly probably requires the formation of adherens junctions [Taniguchi et al, 2005]. In general, expression of the adherens junctions correlated with the desmosomes in well and moderately differentiated HCCs. A substantial number of tumor cells within a given tumor expressed the adherens junctions and the desmosomes simultaneously, but in a few HCCs, particularly in poorly differentiated HCCs, the complementary expression of the adherens junctionsand the desmosomes could be seen.

The expression of the tight junction, symplekin and ZO-1, was not associated with that of the adherens junctions and the desmosomes examined. Symplekin and ZO-1 was especially sensitive in malignant hapatocellular lesions. Many of the tumor cells had apparently lost the ability to express symplekin and ZO-1 in well and moderately differentiated HCCs. Furthermore, almost all cancer cells were negative in poorly differentiated HCCs.

4. Alteration of Cellular Polarity in Hccs

Loss of polarity is an important feature of malignant transformation of colorectal epithelial cell and hepatocyte [Cao et al, 1997; Stamatoglou et al, 1994]. One of signs for the loss of polarity is the apolar distribution of proteins. In normal hepatocytes and benign lesions, β-galactoside α2,6 sialyltransferase was located in the Golgi region surrounding the bile canaliculi, while malignant hepatocyte lesions display diffuse cytoplasm of the tumor cells. Normal hepatocytes expressed CD22 ligand and sialoadhesin ligand at the apical membrane, along the bile canaliculi.

In contrast, the tumor cells strongly expressed ligands for CD22 and sialoadhesin in the Golgi region, in the diffuse cytoplasm, and at the plasma membrane [Cao et al, 2002].

Adhesion molecules are involved in maintaining cellular polarity. The distribution of the adherens junctions and the desmosomes was restricted to the lateral domain of the plasma membrane in normal hepatocytes and benign including probable premalignant lesions, but malignant hepatocyte lesions reveal total plasma membrane, diffuse cytoplasm, and/or even nucleus distribution.

	Junctions	Polarity
Normal hepatocytes	Homogeneous Normal localization	Polarity
Regenerative lesions of hepatocytes	Homogeneous Normal localization	Polarity
Dysplastic lesions and adenoma	Heterogen Slight reduction	Minimal alteration
Well and moderately differentiated hepatocellular carcinoma	Reduction Heterogeneous Alteration of localization	Apolar
Poorly differentiated hepatocellular carcinoma	Strong reduction or loss	Apolar

Figure 1. Alteration of polarity and adhesion molecule in various lesions of the hepatocyte.

The polarity of hepatocytes was associated with the expression of the adherens junctions and desmosomes. Tumor cells with abnormal distribution or loss of the adherens junctions and desmosomes showed an apolar arrangement of tissue architecture [Cao et al, 2007]. In a current study, we observed that decreased expression of symplekin could result in loss of cellular polarity (Chang et al. unpublished data). The relationship of alteration of polarity and adhesion molecules in various lesions of hepatocyteswas shown in figure 1.

5. Pathophysiological Roles of Alteration of Adhesion Molecules Expression and Cellular Polarity

The changes in the expression and cellular distribution of the adhesion molecules as well as the cellular polarity play important roles in development and progression of HCC. (1) Abnormal location and decrease/loss of the adhesion molecules in cancer cells may reduce the adherence of hepatocytes to their neighboring cells. These pathophysiological functions might cause or promote invasive growth of tumor cells. (2) Some adhesion molecules (e.g. β-catenin) are associated with signal transduction and are regularly expressed and distributed at different membrane domains and it is also possible that an abnormal expression and distribution of the adhesion molecules interferes with normal cellular signalling. (3) Adhesion molecules of epithelial cells contribute to maintain cellular polarity. Because of loss of polarity in cancer cells due to reduction of adherence between hepatocytes, other adhesion molecules, e.g. integrins, CD44, could be located anywhere on the cell surface of apolar cancer cells instead of its restricted localization in normal cells and might allow aberrant binding to the extracellular matrix and endothelial cells. (4) The tight junction molecule ZO-1 is homologous to the *Drosophila* discs-large tumor suppressor protein and may be involved in signal transduction and cell proliferation [Willott et al, 1993]. Symplekin, another tight junction molecule, is a multifunctional protein and is involved incomplex functions such as mRNA polyadenylation [Barnard et al, 2004], regulation of the cell cycle [Kavanagh et al, 2006], differentiation of intestinal cells [Buchert et al, 2009], mitosis of cancer cells [Cappell et al, 2010], and tumorigenesis [Buchert et al, 2010]. Tight junctions decreased progressively during rat hepatocarcinogenesis in the previous study [Zhong et al, 1994]. In the current study, we found that an abnormal expression of symplekin was involved in the increased permeability of epithelial monolayersand the change of cellular proliferation in vitro (Chang et al, unpublished data). Taken together, it is tempting to speculate that decreased expression of tight junctions may be an early step in the transformation of a normal hepatocyte. In contrast, decreased expression and abnormal distribution of the adherens junctions and desmosomes may be subject to more serious alteration and lead to further consequences such as causing or promoting the epithelial cells to leave their original site and commence invasive growth.

6. Mechanisms of Alteration of Adhesion Molecules Expression in HCCs

Abnormal expression of E-cadherin and β-catenin has been investigated. Decreased expression of E-cadherin was associated with the loss of one copy of the E-cadherin gene [Slagie et al, 1993], hypermethylation of the E-cadherin promoter [Kanai et al, 1997; Chang et al, 2008], and HBxAg [Liu et al, 2006]. Mechanisms of the abnormal expression of β-catenin were involved in more grounds such as β-catenin gene mutations [de la Coste et al, 1998] and P53 mutations [Cagatay et al, 2002]. The Par3/Par6/aPKC complex which is referred to as polarity proteins and located at the tight junction is required for the tight junction assembly and maintenance, knockdown of Dlg (Discs large) and loss of PALS1 (Protein associated with lin-7) disrupted the adherens junctions formation and E-cadherin locolization [Feigin and Muthuswamy, 2009]. In the current study, we found that decreased expression of symplekinin HCCs was involved in the status of the symplekin promoter and microRNAs (Chang et al, unpublished data). However, studies addressing mechanisms of other adhesion molecules expression are very limited so far.

7. Some Adhesion Moleculescould be used for the Diagnostic approach of HCC

Early diagnosis of HCC, when the prognosis is still favorable, is difficult, because in its early stages it is usually asymptomatic and often coexists with cirrhosis. It has been reported that detecting of carcinoma cells in blood using immunological methods with monoclonal antibodies may be helpful in early detection of carcinomas and in prognosis of metastatic spread. [Racila et al, 1998]. Unlike other solid tumors, many sinusoids can be observed within tumor tissues in early stages of the most of HCCs. Thus, HCC is one of the most suitable types of tumor for application of the immunological methods for early detection. E-cadherin, desmoglein 1, desmoglein 2, desmocollin 2, desmoplakin, and plakophilin 2, are tightly restricted to the epithelial constituents in a normal liver and in various liver diseases, but are completely lacking in hematopoietic and endothelial cells. Thus, these epithelial cell-specific adhesion molecules could be applied as targets to detect carcinoma cells in blood or bone marrow for early detection and prognosis of metastatic spread of HCC. It was known that HCC expressed epithelial cell-associated markers, such as cytokeratin and MUC1 [Cao et al, 1999]. E-cadherin and the above-mentioned desmosomes could be superior to cytokeratin and MUC1, as they are more sensitive.

References

Barnard D.C., Ryan K., Manley J.L., Richter J.D. (2004) *Symplekin and xGLD-2 are required for CPEB-mediated cytoplasmic polyadenylation.* Cell, 119, 641-51.

Birchmeier W. (1995) *E-cadherin as a tumor invasion suppressor gene.* BioEssays, 17, 97-99.

Buchert M., Darido C., Lagerqvist E., Sedello A., Cazevieille C., et al. (2009). *The symplekin/ZONAB complex inhibits intestinal cell differentiation by the repression of AML1/Runx1.* Gastroenterology, 137, 156-64.

Buchert M., Papin M., Bonnans C., Darido C., Raye W.S., et al. (2010) *Symplekin promotes tumorigenicity by up-regulating claudin-2 expression.* Proc Natl Acad Sci USA, 107, 2628-33.

Cagatay T. and Ozturk M. (2002) *P53 mutation as a source of aberrant beta-catenin accumulation in cancer cells.* Oncogene, 21, 7971-7980.

Cao Y., Schlag P.M., Karsten U. (1997) *Immunodetection of epithelial mucin (MUC1, MUC3) and mucin-associated glycotopes (TF, Tn, and Sialosyl-Tn) in benign and malignant lesions of colon epithelium: apolar localization correspond to the malignant transformation.* Virchows Arch, 431, 159-166.

Cao Y., Karsten U., Otto G., Bannasch P. (1999) *Expression of MUC1, Thomsen-Friedenreich antigen, Tn, sialosyl-Tn, and α2,6-linked sialic acid in hepatocellular carcinomas and preneoplastic hepatocellular lesions.* Virchows Arch, 434, 503-509.

Cao Y., Merling A., Crocker P.R., Schwartz-Albiez R. (2002) *Differential Expression of β-galactoside α2,6 sialyltransferase (ST6Gal.I) and sialoglycans in normal and cirrhotic liver and hepatocellular carcinomas.* Lab Invest, 82, 1515-1524.

Cao Y., Chang H., Li L., Cheng R.C., Fan X.N. (2007) *Alteration of adhesion molecule expression and cellular polarity in hepatocellular carcinoma.* Histopathology, 51, 528-38.

Cappell K.M., Larson B., Sciaky N., Whitehurst A.W. (2010) *Symplekin specifies mitotic fidelity by supporting microtubule dynamics.* Mol Cell Biol, 30, 5135-44.

Chang H., Yi B., Li L., Zhang H.Y., Sun F., Dong S.Q., Cao Y. (2008) *Methylation of tumor associated genes in tissue and plasma samples from liver diseases patients*. Exp Mol Pathol, 85, 96-100.

de L Coste A., Romagnolo B., Billuart P., et al. (1998) *Somatic mutations of the β-catenin gene are frequent in mouse and human hepatocellular carcinomas*. Proc Natl Acad Sci UAS, 95, 8847-8851.

Feigin M.E. and Muthuswamy S. (2009) *Polarity proteins regulate mammalian cell-cell junctions and cancer pathogenesis.* Curr Opin Cell Biol, 21, 694-700.

Franke W.W. (2009) *Discovering the molecular components of intercellular junctions—A historical view*. Cold Spring Harb Perspect Biol, 1, a003061.

Furuse M. (2010) *Molecular basis of the core structure of tight junctions.* Cold Spring Harb Perspect Biol, 2, a002907.

Garrod D., Chidgey M., North A. (1996) *Desmosomes: differentiation, development, dynamics and disease.* Curr Opin Cell Biol, 8, 670-678.

Hubbard A.L., Wall D.A., Ma A. (1983) *Isolation of rat hepatocyte plasma membranes. I. Presenence of the three major domains*. J Cell Biol,96, 217-229.

Ihara A., Koizumi H., Hashizume R., Uchikoshi T. (1996) *Expression of epithelial cadherin and□ α- and β-catenin in nontumoral livers and hepatocellular carcinomas*. Hepatology, 23, 1441-1447.

Inagawa S., Itabashi M., Adachi S.,et al. (2002) *Expression and prognostic roles of beta-catenin in hepatocellular carcinoma: correlation with tumor progression and postoperative survival.* Clin Cancer Res, 8, 450-456.

International Working Party (1995) *Terminology of nodular hepatocellular lesions.* Hepatology, 22, 983-993.

Kanai Y., Ushijima S., Hui A.M., et al. (1997) *The E-cadherin gene is silenced by CpG methylation in human hepatochllular carcinomas.* Int J Cancer, 71, 355-359.

Kavanagh E., Buchert M., Tsapara A., Choquet A., Balda M.S., et al. (2006) *Functional interaction between the ZO-1-interacting transcription factor ZONAB/DbpA and the RNA processing factor symplekin*. J Cell Sci, 119, 5098-105.

Keon B.H., Schäfer S., Kuhn C., Grund C., Franke W.W. (1996) *Symplekin, a novel type of tight junction plaque protein.* J Cell Biol, 134, 1003-1018.

Kozyraki R., Scoazec J.Y., Flejou J.F., et al. (1996) *Expression of cadherins and α-catenin in primary epithelial tumors of the liver*. Gastroenterology, 110, 1137-1149.

Lecuit T. (2005) *Adhesion remodeling underlying tissue morphogenesis*. Trend Cell Biol, 15, 34-42.

Liu J., Lian Z., Han S., et al. (2006) *Downregulation of E-cadherin by hepatitis B virus X antigen in hepatocellullar carcinoma*. Oncogene, 25, 1008-10017.

Mertens C., Kuhn C., Franke W.W. (1996) *Plakophilins 2a and 2b: constitutive proteins of dual location in the karyoplasm and the desmosomal plaque*. J Cell Biol, 135, 1009-1025.

Miyoshi Y., Iwao K., Nagasawa Y., et al. (1998) *Activation of the β-catenin gene in primary hepatocellular carcinomas by somatic alterations involving exon 3.* Cancer Res, 58, 2524-2527.

Perl A.K., Wilgenbus P., Dahl U., Semb H., Christofori G. (1998) *A causal role for E-cadherin in the transition from adenoma to carcinoma.* Nature, 392, 190-193.

Racila E., Euhus D., Weiss A.J., et al. (1998) *Detection and characterization of carcinoma cells in the blood.* Proc Natl Acad Sci USA, 95, 4589-4594.

Stamatoglou S.C. and Hughes R.C. (1994) *Cell adhesion molecules in liver function and pattern formation.* FASEB J, 8, 420-427.

Slagie B.L., Zhou Y.Z., Birchmeier W., Scorsone K.A. (1993) *Deletion of the E-cadherin gene in hepatitis B virus-positive chinese hepatocellular carcinomas*. Hepatology, 18, 757-762.

Taniguchi T., Miyazaki M., Miyashita Y., Arima T., Ozawa M. (2005) *Identification of regions of alpha-catenin required for desmosome organization in epithelial cells*. Int Mol Med, 16, 1003-1008.

Wei Y., Van Nhieu J.T., Prigent S., et al. (2002) *Altered expression of E-cadherin in hepatocellular carcinoma: correlations with genetic alterations, beta-catenin expression, and clinical features.* Hepatology, 36, 692-701.

Willott E., Balda M.S., Fanning A.S., Jameson B., Itallie C.V., Anderson J.M. (1993) *The tight junction protein ZO-1 is homologous to the Drosophila discs-large tumor suppressor protein of septate junctions.* Proc Natl Acad Sci UAS, 90, 7834-7838.

Zhang H.Y., Chang H., Fan X.N., Zhang K.D., Yu L., Cao Y. (2011) *Expression of adhesion molecules and mucins in human and rhesus macaque gastrointestinal epithelial cells.* Histol Histopathol, 26, 1405-1413.

Zhong Y., Enomoto K., Tobika H., Konishi Y., Satoh M., Mori M. (1994) *Sequential decrease in tight junctions as revealed by 7H6 tight junction-associated protein during rat hepatocarcinogenesis.* Jpn J Cancer Res, 85, 351-356.

In: Liver Disease and Peritonitis
Editor: Mao Kang Voung et al.
ISBN 978-1-61942-080-9

Chapter 6

Peritonitis: Symptoms, Treatment and Prevention

***Neha Salvi*[1] *and Sachchidananda Maiti*[2]**
[1]Speciality Trainee, Obstetrics and Gynaecology,
North Manchester General Hospital, Manchester, UK
[2]Consultant in Obstetrics and Gynaecology,
North Manchester General Hospital, Manchester, UK

Abstract

The inflammation of the peritoneum, a mesothelial membrane, is referred to as peritonitis.

The most common cause of peritonitis is bacterial contamination. The other causes are tuberculosis, Chlamydia, fungi, chemical, biliary, drugs and foreign body. Peritonitis can be differentiated into primary, secondary and tertiary.

The most common symptom with which the patient presents is pain which can be localized or generalised. Associated symptoms may include anorexia, nausea, vomiting and malaise. Patients may also present with systemic inflammatory response with fever, tachycardia and tachypnoea. Some patients may present in septic or hypovolemic shock. Tenderness, guarding and rebound tenderness are present on abdominal examination. Bowel sounds are either diminished or absent.

The aim of the treatment is to restore the fluid and electrolyte balance, provide support to the organs and control the source of infection. Initial management is to control the pain, fluid resuscitation, appropriate broad spectrum antibiotics intravenously and oxygen. Definitive management is surgery and should not be delayed except for certain cases like acute pancreatitis. Surgical treatment is mainly laparotomy, though it may be possible to manage some cases by laparoscopy. The aim is to control the source of infection by resection or closure, draining abscesses, removing debris and necrotic tissues by lavage or debridement.

Most cases of peritonitis cannot be prevented. It is possible to reduce the incidence of peritonitis in specific cases. Long term antibiotic prophylaxis is proven to reduce the incidence of spontaneous bacterial peritonitis in patients with cirrhosis. Incidence of peritonitis can be reduced in patients on continuous ambulatory dialysis by measures to prevent the invasion of bacteria through or around the lumen of the catheter. Taking steps to avoid the rupture of dermoid cyst during surgery will prevent cases of chemical peritonitis.

Keywords: antibiotics, bacteria, catheter, laparotomy, peritonitis, prevention, shock, surgery, tenderness

Introduction

The inflammation of peritoneum, a mesothelial membrane, is referred to as peritonitis. Inflammatory reaction of the peritoneum may be secondary to infection, injury or irritation and results in exudates in the peritoneal cavity [1]

Aetiology

Bacterial peritonitis is the most common cause of peritonitis and is further classified into Primary, secondary and tertiary. Chemical or aseptic peritonitis accounts for about 20% of the cases in the UK. It is secondary to a perforated duodenal or gastric ulcer. Progression to secondary bacterial peritonitis occurs within a few hours due to transmigration of organisms e.g. from the bowel.[2]

Other forms of sterile peritonitis are biliary, due to pancreatic juices, blood, urine and meconium. Chlamydial peritonitis: Chlamydia is a common cause of pelvic inflammatory disease leading to peritonitis. Foreign bodies like talc and starch from the surgical gloves can lead to inflammatory response in the peritoneum. Drugs: intra-peritoneal chemotherapy can lead to clinical symptoms resembling acute peritonitis.

Tuberculous Peritonitis

It is rare in the developed economy countries and mainly seen in immigrant population or in immunocompromised patients in western world. The spread to the peritoneum can be blood borne or direct spread from lymph nodes, bowel or tuberculous pyosalpinx.

Classification

Peritonitis can be differentiated into primary, secondary and tertiary [3]

In primary peritonitis there is no breach of the gastrointestinal tract and no source from within the abdomen which can be identified. Examples are spontaneous bacterial peritonitis typically seen in patients with cirrhosis of liver and patients on continuous ambulatory peritoneal dialysis for chronic renal failure with an indwelling intra-peritoneal catheter. Other rare causes are streptococcal peritonitis in young females and accidental puncture of gastrointestinal tract during paracentesis.

The most frequent form of peritonitis is secondary peritonitis which is as a result of a local infectious process within the peritoneal cavity. It can occur in the presence or absence of perforation of a hollow viscus and lead to diffuse peritonitis. Tertiary peritonitis is a persistent or recurrent peritonitis occurring at least 48hrs after the apparent adequate management of primary or secondary peritonitis. It may occur when the source control is unsuccessful, antimicrobial treatment is ineffective or due to immunosuppression [4]

Clinical Presentation

Symptoms

The most common presenting symptom is generalised or localised abdominal pain. The pain caused due to visceral perforation initially presents as a sharp sudden onset pain mainly in the area of perforation but may become more generalised as the peritoneal contamination spreads. There may be referred pain to the shoulder tip. Other associated symptoms are fever, malaise, anorexia and vomiting. Diarrhoea may be presenting symptom in case of pelvic abscess.

Patients with tuberculous peritonitis may present with acute symptoms as above. The onset can be chronic with symptoms of long standing abdominal pain, night sweats, weight loss, fever and abdominal distensions. Pelvic tuberculosis may present in females with pelvic mass, subfertility, abnormal bleeding and pelvic pain.

Signs

The patient will appear to be anxious, pale with sunken eyes due to dehydration. The observations will show signs of systemic inflammatory response with fever, tachycardia and tachypnoea. The patient may present in septic shock with fever or hypothermia, hypotension, tachycardia and tachypnoea. The patient will lie relatively motionless in supine position with the knees flexed. The respirations are usually rapid and shallow.

Abdominal palpation will elicit tenderness, rebound tenderness and rigidity due to spasm of the abdominal muscles. Initially the tenderness will be at the site of pathology later there will be generalised signs. The bowel sounds may be sluggish or absent due to ileus.

Ascites is present in more than 90% of the patients with tuberculous peritonitis at the time of presentation, the remainder may present with a more advanced dry phase which represents a fibroadhesive form of disease (classic doughy abdomen).[5,6].

Treatment

Major generalised peritonitis is associated with multi-organ failure and a high mortality. The treatment will depend on the cause of peritonitis.The main principles of treatment are restoration of the fluid and electrolyte imbalance; provide physiological support to the organs, appropriate broad spectrum antimicrobial treatment and control the source of infection. [7]

The peritoneal cavity has a large surface area and inflammation results in sequestration of large volumes of fluid. This and associated symptoms of vomiting or diarrhoea can lead to fluid and electrolyte imbalance. The initial fluid replacement is with intravenous crystalloids, amount will depend on degree of shock. Electrolyte supplement may be required depending on result of the blood electrolytes levels.

Failing organ systems will need support to be restored to the normal state. High flow oxygen is vital for patients presenting with shock. Hypoxia should be monitored. These patients will require monitoring of the central venous pressures to help guide the fluid administration. Those presenting in shock or with hypotension will need ionotropes.

An important adjunct for the treatment is prompt initiation of broad spectrum (covers aerobes and anaerobes) antimicrobial treatment intravenously, ideally within 3 hours of emergency admission as per the Sepsis 6 hour care bundle.[8]. Early and appropriate treatment will prevent the local and haematogenous spread and reduce late complications and mortality.

The duration of the treatment will depend on the type of infection, host immunity and the response to the treatment. The generally recommended duration is 5-7 days; it can be safely stopped after the clinical resolution of the symptoms [9]. A longer duration of treatment of up to 10-14 days may be longer in patients who are more unwell and have generalised peritonitis.

Recommended antimicrobial agents [10] from the surgical infection society for treatment of peritonitis are as follows:

Single Agents

Ampicillin/sulbactam
Cefotetan
Cefoxitin
Ertapenem
Imipenem/cilastatin
Meropenem
Piperacillin/tazobactam
Ticarcillin/clavulanic acid

Combination Regimens

Aminoglycoside (amikacin, gentamicin, netilmicin, tobramycin) plus an antianaerobe
Aztreonam plus clindamycin
Cefuroxime plus metronidazole
Ciprofloxacin plus metronidazole
Third/fourth-generation cephalosporin (cefepime, cefotaxime, ceftazidime, ceftizoxime, ceftriaxone) plus an antianaerobe.

No specific recommendations can be made for the first line treatment of secondary peritonitis in adults with antibiotics, as all regimens showed equivocal efficacy. Other factors such as local guidelines and preferences ease of administration, costs and availability must therefore be taken into consideration in deciding the antibiotic regimen of choice. Future trials should attempt to stratify patients and perform intention-to-treat analysis to allow better external validity (Cochrane review).[11]

Conservative or medical management is indicated in cases where the infection has localised, in cases of acute pancreatitis, if patient is not fit for surgery. These patients are managed with intra venous fluids, broad spectrum antimicrobial agents and support to other organ systems.

Surgical treatment in form of laparotomy should not be delayed if surgery is indicated. Delay in operative management is associated with increased mortality. The objectives of surgery are to find the cause of peritonitis and control the source of infection. Source control is the interventions which eliminate the focus of infection, control the ongoing contamination and restore the normal anatomy and function. The control of primary source of sepsis requires managing the source of contamination by resection or closure, draining the abscesses, debriding the necrotic tissue and removal of debris and faecal material. [12]

The evidence for clinical benefit of peritoneal lavage is little. It may be possibly due to the resistance of the microbial peritoneal cavities to lavage adequately, or due to the concomitant damage to the mesothelial cells caused by peritoneal irrigation.

Conclusion

Clinical outcome in peritonitis is dependent on several factors -cause, effectiveness of antimicrobial agent, timing of diagnosis and commencement of remedial actions. The controversy still remains on optimal duration of antibiotic treatment and effective measures for minimising intra peritoneal adhesion formation.

References

[1] Wittmann DH, Schein M, Condon RE. Management of secondary peritonitis. *Ann. Surg.* 1996; 224: 10-8.

[2] Skipworth RJE, Feron KCH. Acute abdomen: peritonitis.emergency. *Surgery* 2007;26:3, 98-101.

[3] Blot S, Waele J De .Critical issues in the clinical management of complicated intra- abdomional infections. *Drugs* 2005;65(12)1611-1620.

[4] Malangoni MA. Evaluation and management of tertiary peritonitis. *Am. Surg.* 2000;66:157– 61.

[5] Manohar, A, Simjee, AE, Haffejee, AA, Pettengell, KE. Symptoms and investigative findings in 145 patients with tuberculous peritonitis diagnosed by peritoneoscopy and biopsy over a five year period. *Gut* 1990; 31:1130.

[6] Bhargava, DK, Shriniwas, Chopra, P, Nijhawan, et al. Peritoneal tuberculosis: laparoscopic patterns and its diagnostic accuracy. *Am. J. Gastroenterol.* 1992; 87:109.

[7] Malangoni MA. Contributions to the management of intraabdominal infections. *Am. J. Surg.* 2005;190:255-59.

[8] Surviving sepsis campaign management guidelines committee. Guidelines on management of severe sepsis and septic shock. *Crit. care med.* 2004;32:3.

[9] Solomkin JS, Mazuski JE, Baron EJ, et al. Guidelines for the selection of anti-infective agents for complicated intra-abdominal infections. *Clin. Infect Dis.* 2003; 37: 997-1005.

[10] Mazuski J E, Sawyer R G, Nathens A B, Dipiro JT, Schein M et al The Surgical Infection Society Guidelines on Antimicrobial Therapy for Intra-Abdominal Infections: An Executive Summary. *Surgical Infections* 2002;3(3):165.

[11] Antibiotic regimens for secondary peritonitis of gastrointestinal origin in adults 2008(4).

[12] Deveney CW, Lurie K, Deveney KE. Improved treatment of intra abdominal abscess. A result of improved localization, drainage, and patient care, not technique. *Arch. Surg.* 1988;123:1126 –30.

Index

A

D

E

I

J

K

L

M

N

O

P

Q

R

S

T

U

V

W

Y